beyond childlessness

FOR EVERY WOMAN WHO EVER WANTED TO HAVE A CHILD – AND DIDN'T

Rachel Black & Louise Scull

RODALE

This edition first published in 2005 by
Rodale International Ltd
7–10 Chandos Street
London
W1G 9AD
www.rodale.co.uk

Book design by Briony Chappell

Printed and bound in the UK by CPI Bath using acid-free paper from sustainable sources.

1 3 5 7 9 8 6 4 2

A CIP record for this book is available from the British Library.

ISBN 1-4050-7761-1

This paperback edition distributed to the book trade by Pan Macmillan Ltd.

Notice
This book is intended as a reference volume only, not as a medical manual. The information given here is designed to help you make informed decisions about your health. It is not intended as a substitute for any treatment that may have been prescribed by your doctor. If you suspect that you have a medical problem, we urge you to seek competent medical help.

Mention of specific companies, organizations or authorities in this book does not imply endorsement by the publisher, nor does mention of specific companies, organizations or authorities in the book imply that they endorse this book.

Addresses, websites and telephone numbers given in this book were accurate at the time it went to press.

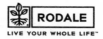

RODALE
LIVE YOUR WHOLE LIFE™

We inspire and enable people to improve their lives and the world around them

Contents

Acknowledgements

We would like to thank everyone who has helped to turn the idea of *Beyond Childlessness* into a reality.

In particular, we would like to thank all of you who agreed to be interviewed for your courage and honesty in sharing so generously your time, your stories and all your emotions with us – you know who you are, and without you, this book would never have been written.

To the health-care professionals, thank you for taking us seriously, and for giving us the benefit of your time and your expertise.

To everyone who helped put us in touch with the women we interviewed, particularly where this involved venturing into uncharted territory, thank you for your belief in us and for being prepared to break the taboo.

To our partners and friends, thank you for putting up with our single-minded obsession over the last 2 years, and also for positively encouraging and supporting us when the going got tough.

To Anne, Susannah, Adrian, Helen and Liz at Rodale, thank you for your unflagging enthusiasm and support, and finally to Leslee – without your belief in us, your advice and all your efforts on our behalf, *Beyond Childlessness* could never have happened.

Introduction

'Do you have children?'

My heart sinks. When I answer 'No, actually I don't', what response will I get?

'Don't worry, you've got plenty of time yet' (actually, that's not true, I'm 46).

Or, 'You don't know how lucky you are, not having children' (and you don't know how I feel about not having children, so how can you say such a thing).

Or, perhaps, 'You can borrow mine any time you like' (that's not really the point, is it).

Or, if you're single, that old favourite 'When you meet Mr Right, then you'll change your mind...'.

Or, perhaps even worse, the non-committal 'Oh, really', leaving me to speculate on what you're thinking – 'She's selfish, self-centred, immature, unfeminine, cold, a workaholic, materialistic, overly ambitious, unfulfilled...'.

Worst of all, you might actually feel sorry for me.

These are Louise's responses; I (Rachel), after some negotiation with Douglas, now answer the first question with 'No, my husband didn't want any', which is true, and is a truth that I've finally come to accept. It feels OK.

And if you're reading this book, you've probably developed your own way of dealing with this potential conversational minefield. Perhaps your response is, like another friend of ours, 'No, I wanted to spend my money at Conran, not Mothercare'.

But why is it, when so many of us, for a whole host of different reasons, are remaining childless, that we find this subject so difficult to talk about, other than flippantly, vaguely or not at all?

Whether it is a positive choice, or is a result of circumstances, remaining childless is a situation that is rarely without emotional consequences. These may range from an occasional sense of loss, or guilt, perhaps triggered by other people's reactions, to an acute and profound daily sense of grief, with debilitating results.

Helen, one of the many women we talked to for this book, is married and has thought a lot about her childlessness. She is now basically at peace with it; however, she recognises that it touches on all aspects of her life:

I feel as if I've arrived, I say I've arrived, I know I'm at a place but I know that I'm still on a journey, and so I feel now that I'm able to say 'Look, it can be really fun, you can make it worth while, you can still find value in your life, you might have to do it differently but you can'. But I think that's on the back of quite a lot of hard work, to be honest, a lot of hard work in a lot of areas. I think childlessness touches on lots of things – it's almost like a big bowl of spaghetti, and you're going to take quite a long time to sort out that bowl of spaghetti, and see how it touches – it does touch things like your relationship with your mum, your relationship with your sisters if you've got any, your friends, your work, your career, how all the bits of the jigsaw fit together. I think that just takes a long time to evolve, and you don't have all the answers at the beginning.

About us

We met on holiday on the island of Skyros, Greece, almost 5 years ago. At the time, we were both living and working in London, both struggling with getting better work–life balance, and when we came back from the holiday it was natural to stay in touch, meeting up for the occasional drink. As we got to know each other better, we inevitably shared more of our stories and were struck by some of the similarities in our past experiences.

One of the things that Rachel shared was the story of her childlessness, and her idea, at that stage unfulfilled, for writing a book to help other women learning to live with childlessness. Louise, struck by the power of this idea, suggested a collaboration, and the idea for this book was born.

Although we have both studied and taken part in various types of therapy, we are not social workers, health workers or professional psychologists. Our main 'qualification' for writing this book is that we are both childless women and, as such, we feel it is important to share our own stories and experiences here too.

As you will see from our stories on pages 18 and 20, we represent different ends of the spectrum of childless women. The many women we have interviewed for this project represent all points in between. Every story is different, yet there are common themes, particularly in the emotional roller-coaster of our experiences, and in the variety of coping strategies we have adopted.

About the women we talked to

In researching this book, we talked to over 200 childless women, from many different backgrounds and cultures, ranging in age from their early 30s to well into their 70s. We also carried out in-depth interviews with many of these women and a handful of men who expressed a strong desire to talk about their childlessness. We also talked to a number of female professionals, primarily counsellors in the fields of infertility, adoption, surrogacy and psychosexuality, who are all very experienced in helping women with issues around childlessness.

The women we interviewed had a variety of reasons for remaining childless – infertility (their own, their partner's or unexplained), early menopause, leaving it too late, not finding the right partner at the right time, being with a partner who doesn't want children – the stories are rarely straightforward. They include a number of women who have had one or more children, and desperately wanted more. About half of the women have chosen to appear in this book under their real names, with the rest choosing to use a fictional name.

But the stories are real, as are the words, and the emotions.

As Dr Rachel Naomi Remen says, in her book *Kitchen Table Wisdom: Stories That Heal*:

> All stories are full of bias and uniqueness; they mix fact with meaning. This is the root of their power. Stories allow us to see something familiar through new eyes. We become in that moment a guest in someone else's life, and together with them sit at the feet of their teacher. The meaning we may draw from someone else's story may be different from the meaning they themselves have drawn. No matter. Facts bring us to knowledge, but stories lead to wisdom.

Childlessness – the facts and figures

Across the developed world, the birth rate is falling consistently. In the UK, the average number of births per woman is now 1.64, the lowest level since records began in 1924, and only just over half the rate of the 'baby boom' 40 years ago. In New Zealand, the average number of births per woman is now just over 2.0, in Australia, the average is 1.75 and, in South Africa, the average for the white population is 1.8. In continental Europe, rates are even lower, averaging between 1.3 and 1.5 births per woman. In total across the developed world, more than 60 countries, including the USA, now have birth rates that are below replacement level – i.e. lower than 2.1 births per woman.

Rates of childlessness are also increasing, although this does not directly correlate with birth rates, due to differences in the average size of family in different countries. For example, Spain has the lowest birth rate in Europe, at around 1.2, but also has a relatively low level of childlessness, with only 11 per cent of Spanish women not having children. The rates for Japan are very similar, and research shows that most developed countries have rates of childlessness in the range 10–15 per cent.

Rates of childlessness are particularly high in the UK and the USA, where estimates are that 20–25 per cent of women who are currently of childbearing age will in fact remain childless. In Australia, recent projections by the Australian Institute of Family Studies suggest that as many as 28 per cent of young Australian women will remain childless, with the figure projected to be as high as 33 per cent in some states. In New Zealand, the latest census figures show a 14 per cent increase in the number of childless women over the past 15 years.

In all these countries, childlessness is not spread evenly across the population as a whole, but is particularly pronounced among career women and women with higher levels of educational achievement. A recent Australian study on lifetime childlessness, for example, showed that women who have an undergraduate degree or higher level qualification are more than twice as likely to be childless as their peers without such qualifications. A recent study based on census data in the UK shows that 59 per cent of female managers do not have children, compared to only 29 per cent of their male colleagues (Rosemary Crompton, Leicester University). Interestingly, at the time of writing, of the 118 women Members of Parliament in the UK House of Commons, 41, or 35 per cent, are childless.

But are these high levels of childlessness through choice, or through force of circumstances? A recent study by the Family Policy Studies Centre shows that only 11 per cent of British women actually plan to remain childless, whereas more than twice this number will actually do so.

Infertility is part of the explanation for this difference – as many as one in six couples may have problems conceiving, with a total of approximately 600,000 infertile couples in the UK. Somewhere between 30,000 and 40,000 UK couples each year consult their GP with concerns about fertility. This represents an increase of over 50 per cent in the past five years, although this is likely to be as much a reflection of increased awareness of fertility treatments as of any actual increase in infertility.

The trend across the developed world is certainly towards women having their first child later in life than would previously have been the case. In the UK, the average age for a woman having her first child rose from 26.4 years to 29 years over the last quarter of the 20th century; over a similar period in the USA, the average age for a woman having her first child rose from 21.4 years to 25 years. In both countries, although not statistically quantified, the figure would clearly be much higher for middle-class women with careers.

With advances in assisted reproductive technology such as IVF, and high profile cases of older women, some post-menopausal, successfully having children, it is tempting to think that we can put off having children until our careers are successfully established. However, IVF treatment alone is not particularly effective for women over the age of 40. There is only about a 10 per cent pregnancy success rate, with a significantly higher risk of miscarriage than for younger mothers. IVF using donor eggs has a better success rate – around 20–25 per cent measured in terms of live births – but that still means that the failure rate is 75–80 per cent. Many women, as illustrated by some of the stories in this book, may find that they have literally left it too late, either in terms of finding a partner or, if they have a partner, in terms of being able to conceive.

The conspiracy of silence

What came as a real surprise to us was how few of the women we interviewed had actually talked about their stories before. Even close friends, whom we have known for 20 years or more, have their own stories about their childlessness, of which we were unaware.

On reflection, it's perhaps not so unexpected – as the stories in this book demonstrate; for many women being childless goes to the core of their identity, touching deep and painful emotions. And we all have our own defence mechanisms for dealing with potentially painful conversations – whether it's humour, vagueness, changing the subject – they all have the effect of pushing people away from us, rather than inviting further discussion.

In an age where nothing seems too personal to be discussed, the subject of childlessness isn't talked about, or written about, or in the public domain in any way. It's all too easy to feel that you are the only woman in the world who is struggling with this issue.

And many of us are professional, well-educated women, who are used to being self-sufficient, so we feel we ought to be able to deal with it and move on. This woman's experience following the death of her baby, quoted in DeFrain et al.'s *Sudden Infant Death*, is not unusual:

> Generally during this time I was alone, and eight months after the death of our son, I went into a depression. I didn't move for a month. My husband made supper most of the time. I couldn't feel anything. I probably needed professional help at that point, but neither my husband nor I knew what was wrong or what to expect. Was this normal grief? I thought of the mental health clinic. What would I say if I went there? I'm not an alcoholic. I haven't attempted suicide. I just needed to talk about my baby. Do people go to a mental health office because they have no one to talk to? I didn't know. Besides, I am an intelligent, educated person; I should be able to handle this, I was taught self-sufficiency early. Also, as a Christian, isn't my faith supposed to be enough? Don't I have enough faith? If I do, and I thought I did, I should find God's strength sufficient. If I don't, where do I go with that answer?

While we have been working on the book, there have started to be a few examples of well-known women talking openly about their childlessness (such as Hilary Mantel's autobiography, *Giving Up the Ghost*), although these are still outnumbered by what feels like at least a thousand to one by 'miracle baby' stories, of older women, often post-menopausal, finally having their longed-for child. We really hope that more women will choose to break the conspiracy of silence surrounding childlessness: the more we can listen to other people's stories, and talk of our own feelings, the more we can learn to accept those feelings and to live with our childlessness.

Who this book is for

This book is principally aimed at women aged 35+ who are learning to live with being childless. By sharing childless women's stories, including our own, by looking at our reasons for wanting children and our experiences of remaining childless, and by looking at the emotional consequences of being childless, we want to bring these issues out into the open, and help women acknowledge, understand and accept their feelings. By sharing the different ways women have dealt with being childless, and by providing much-needed role models, we provide practical examples of learning to live with being childless.

The book may also be helpful to younger women who are ambivalent about having children, to partners, family and friends of childless women, to health professionals involved in the support of childless women and to women of all ages who would have liked to have more children.

Perhaps what we are trying to achieve is best summed up by this quote from a recent play by Alan Bennett, *The History Boys*:

> *The best moments in reading are when you come across something – a thought, a feeling, a way of looking at things – which you thought special and particular to you. Now here it is, set down by someone else, a person you may have never met (...) and it is as if a hand has come out and taken yours.*

Rachel's story
I met my husband, Douglas, in a bar in Verbier, Switzerland, during a spur of the moment skiing holiday to celebrate my decision to set up in business as a market research consultant.

Our chance meeting was not love at first sight, but we both felt a deep sense of warmth and belonging which soon blossomed into passion. After the angst surrounding my previous long-term relationships, life with Douglas was fun and totally satisfying. He was everything I wanted and needed in a man. He was warm, funny, intelligent, loving and very proud of, never threatened by, my highly lucrative business. Dating was exciting and fulfilling. We made a fantastic team, admiring and nurturing in each other the skills we lacked in ourselves. I could not believe my luck!

Douglas made it clear from the outset that he never wanted to marry. While I knew I did, I found the situation strangely liberating. Having lived through two failed engagements, I was in no hurry to commit to a third. Instead, I vowed I'd stay with him only as long as I felt happy and fulfilled.

Then six months into the relationship, without any warning, he proposed. It was the happiest day of my life. Firmly believing you only get what you want through effort and application, I remember feeling a touch guilty that our relationship had been so effortless, so easy. My smugness was soon shaken and then shattered, as it slowly dawned on me that the price was phenomenal. This wonderfully clever, strong, witty, talented man I had married did not want children.

I believed that if you're happily married, healthy and financially sound, children are the natural corollary. Before we married, I had talked briefly to Douglas about my desire for children and he'd said nothing to hint at the trauma to come, nothing to intimate he was not fully supportive of my dream of having two little Blacks.

The first inkling I had that my dreams did not match my husband's came a couple of months after our wedding, as we looked for a matrimonial home. It became apparent that for my husband a nursery or playroom was not a priority. When I raised the subject, there was initially evasion, followed by apparent disinterest, which I found a touch annoying, nothing more. There followed about four months of false hopes, accompanied by a growing sense of unease.

Finally, on another skiing holiday almost a year to the day after we first met, I had come to the point where not knowing for sure how my husband felt about having children had become unbearable. Patience had never been one of my strong points. So there, in the small, wooden, thin walled bedroom of the chalet, I confronted him. I wanted a straight answer to a simple question. He gave it to me and I knew at once from the tone and seriousness of his voice that it was his final word on the subject. He'd said 'No children'. Those were the only two words I heard and they broke my heart.

I can remember a weird sound coming from me. It was a strangled primeval scream. In that moment of deepest despair, I was aware that our friends were in the next room, and I didn't want to make a scene or let the side down. It was as if deeply learnt behaviour took over from a mind that had completely flipped.

I spent the next few months in a state of complete shock. I threw myself into my job, work giving me a sense of stability and sanity totally lacking in my relationship. My impulse was to run as far away from Douglas as I could. It was so very painful to be around him. I had to live with the realisation that if I had known that he did not want children, I would never have married him. The price would have been too high for me.

Looking back, there were a few months of marital bliss, followed by five years of heartache. The stress on our marriage was enormous and the recovery process has been long and tortuous. I searched extensively, but could find no book, no magazine article, nothing on coping with childlessness. I believe this total absence of information and support resulted in my taking far longer to cope with my situation and to learn how to move on. I found the lack of any dialogue in the public domain very isolating.

For me, the breakthrough came during therapy when I realised I needed to mourn the children I would never have. It took me years to understand this, but as soon as I did, I no longer felt 'stuck' and was finally able to begin to move on from the great sadness that had engulfed my life.

We've been married now for 16 years, and I feel my life is pretty much back on track. Most of the time, I feel self-confident, fulfilled and content, yet for many years I would not have believed this possible as I struggled to cope with a gaping void that threatened to consume me and my marriage.

Louise's story

I never really thought much about having children when I was young. I felt like the 9-year-old narrator of Evelyn Rosser's story, when she says, 'I don't want a baby. I want a mink coat, a red convertible and a big house on the beach.'

When I was born in 1959, my older sisters were 4½, 7 and 8½, and we lived in a small, semi-detached house in the West Country. My father worked long hours, seven days a week, as a taxi driver, and in my childhood memories of my mother she seemed permanently tired and stressed.

I knew, from a very early age, that I never wanted to live like that, that the most important thing to me was financial (and emotional) independence. Despite some rebellious times during my teens, I did well at school, went to Oxford University and then started work in the City.

When I was 25, I became pregnant as a result of a faulty condom. Even though I was in a good relationship at the time, with someone I loved very much and imagined spending the rest of my life with, it was still a relatively easy decision – I had an abortion. We were too young; we weren't ready to settle down yet; I needed to establish my career first; there was plenty of time.

The relationship didn't last. Perhaps the fact that we never really talked about the abortion, and what it meant to both of us, didn't help.

When I was 35, I became pregnant again, this time as a result of one night with an old flame. Now, it was a much tougher decision. The first decision was whether I should even tell him. After all, we weren't in a relationship, it would be my decision, and whatever that decision was, I wouldn't be looking to him for anything.

In the end, I decided that I would tell him, and I was very glad that I did. One of the things that we hadn't covered in our catching up of news that night was the fact that his recent divorce was at least in part due to the extra stresses and strains placed on the marriage by many months of IVF treatment. Until my call to tell him that I was pregnant, he believed that he might never be able to have children. (He's now happily married again, with three children.)

He was very supportive, told me that he would back me, whatever my decision, and offered to support me financially if I decided to go ahead and have the child. In some ways, this probably made the decision more difficult – I didn't have the excuse that I couldn't afford to be a single parent. And, given my age, and the fact that I wasn't in a relationship, I knew that this might be my last chance to have a child.

After talking to many people, at length, about the options, I decided to have an abortion – I just didn't feel that I could cope, emotionally, with being a single mum.

I'm now 46 and, having recently been diagnosed as post-menopausal, I accept that I will never have children. Despite this, I don't regret either of my decisions, and I know that, faced with the same situations again, I would make the same choices.

But there are still times when it hurts. Until my recent diagnosis, I might see a story in the newspaper about a woman having her first child at the age of 45+, and my heart would leap, as for an instant I thought, 'Ooh, maybe it's not too late after all'. I have three god-children who are very important to me and there are many other children that I spend time with in my life. But it's not the same.

And, just occasionally, I also think forward to old age. As Rachel and I were starting out on this project, I got a telephone call from my mother (then 76) in the middle of the day (she never normally calls before 6 p.m.), asking if I could go down and stay with her for a couple of days, as she was feeling very unwell. After I'd finished talking to her and put the phone down, I couldn't help wondering who I would call in 30 years' time.

And I also recognise that deciding not to have children has given me the freedom to do many other things – not least, to sell my house and give up work almost four years ago, spending a couple of years travelling and sailing, then working on this book with Rachel – none of which would have been possible if I had a child.

But I still can't help wondering if I'll come to regret my decision ...

CHAPTER 1

Wanting a child – the dream

As one speaker at a recent conference on infertility said – if having a child is a major life event, then wanting a child and not being able to have one is a personal life crisis. Recognising the enormous and multi-faceted nature of our dreams of having children, and therefore the enormous and multi-faceted nature of our loss, can be an important part of understanding and learning to live with the pain of being childless.

Early assumptions

For many of us, having children formed an important part of our early childhood dreams. Getting married and having children is not a decision that we might or might not take at some point in the future, but is for most of us an automatic assumption.

It had never occurred to Lara that she might not have children:

As a child growing up, out of the three of us, I was the one that everyone saw as the homemaker with my 2.2 children. I was expected to have the big family, because I liked being in the kitchen, and I looked after people, that kind of thing. So that was the expectation, which is probably what made it even worse, I think, because it never occurred to me I wouldn't.

Some of us build up very detailed pictures of our husbands and children, including the number of children, their sexes, even their names. I (Rachel) can't recall a time when I didn't assume I'd have children. Playing at being mummy, keeping house, naming and caring for dolls, I understood from a very early age I was practising being a mum.

I wanted a boy and a girl. I was always toying with names. I remember wanting unusual names, names that stood out without being embarrassing, like I wanted my children to be. For years, I veered between Harriet and Miriam, Wilfred and Rufus. The only uncertainty in my mind was whether they'd suit my married name!

Clare C's dreams were equally detailed:

I'm a very maternal person. I can remember as a child lying on the sofa pretending to have babies, when I was a little girl, about 5. Always in my mind I had a vision of being a farmer's wife and having four children, and being surrounded by dogs and cats. The dogs and cats thing, and living on the farm, I have fulfilled, but not the having children aspect. I was always very maternal – caring, protective of little things, loving by nature, wanting my own children. It was my ambition to be a farmer's wife with two boys and two girls.

For some of us, like Sally, these early childhood dreams come from a desire or an expectation that we will replicate our own happy childhoods:

I had a happy childhood, and nice parents. In my circle there were very few, I mean virtually no, dysfunctional families, or ghastly kids, and very few divorces. So, generally speaking, I would want to have replicated that, just to be the same as everybody else. And so I wouldn't say I always assumed that I would have children, as I never took it for granted at all, but I always knew that I wanted children.

Following the birth of her daughter when she was 35, Penny B and her husband spent five years trying unsuccessfully to have more children. For Penny, having an only child was not what she had dreamt of, nor expected:

I'm one of three, I have two brothers. I was the eldest, and had always assumed that I'd have three children. I just had this picture, that's what I would be, that's what a family was. It was a very happy family.

And many of us carry these dreams through into adolescence, continuing to live out our dreams through 'parenting' younger siblings, or friends' and neighbours' children. Rebecca B has wanted to have children for as long as she can remember:

One of our neighbours had a baby and I was mad about her; I used to love rocking her and singing to her, which probably wasn't very nice for the child! I would go into bookshops and look at children's books and think how lovely it will be when I can buy these for my own children. And kids' shoes, I always had a complete thing about babies' shoes.

As Alison Bagshawe, Senior Fertility Counsellor at the Assisted Conception Unit of Guy's Hospital, says:

It's can be hard, because there is just so much investment in having a child and it really is just such a fundamental part of most women's lives. People grow up with the assumption that they will get pregnant. It is locked so deep into most female psyche to be a mother. It's like they weave a tapestry throughout their life and each experience, each part fills in more of it, more of the picture that it's going to be. Then when they are told or realise that this is not going to happen, they are left with all the work and the tapestry that cannot be undone. I'm talking about maybe 30 or 40 years of experience, of their fantasies of how they're going to be as a mother, recreating their own childhood, making it better for their own child, giving a son to the family – there are so many parts to this that it's like weaving this tapestry and you cannot unpick it. It is what has made up the essential fibre of a person.

Some people weave this really intricate tapestry, and it's so complicated, so full of things. Some people are more able to deal with it because they haven't put so much into it, they're more able to move on and out.

Having it all

Although our dreams may have been very detailed, for a significant proportion of us a husband and children were only part of our expectations. Unlike many of our mothers' generation, we expected to 'have it all' – a successful career, and a happy marriage and children. And although many of us planned our careers and other aspects of our lives in meticulous detail, we didn't actually plan for our children – we just assumed that children would happen, that they would automatically fall into place when the time was right. I (Rachel) saw children as a rite of passage between puberty and the menopause, part of the natural rhythm of life – birth, life, renewal and decay, a fundamental life stage I wanted to experience when I was mature but not old.

Sarah A is a very successful management consultant in her mid-40s:

Leaving university, wanting to support myself, that's always been a given, I think. It wasn't that I was a feminist, anti-men, anti-children, anything like that, it's just that I left university with a good qualification, got into a good job, why wouldn't you? In fact, I felt beholden – you have a good degree, you don't go and get married and have children straight away and throw it all away. I expected to get married, to have children, to be supported, not subservient, to have a career, but to stop my career to have children for a while and then probably blossom into a career in later life.

But the idea of having children in our 20s or early 30s, our time of peak fertility, clashes with our career aspirations and may also be a time when we are more concerned with establishing our identity as an adult, and as a woman, rather than thinking about our identity as a mother. As Sarah A goes on to say:

I do remember (in my late 20s) one girlfriend, a little older than me, married, leaving work to have a baby, and me thinking wistfully 'Yes, I want to do that, but not yet, I don't want to give up on my education, the job I've got'.

As time goes on, it can become increasingly difficult to work out how to have it all – to continue with a successful career and at the same time establish a family. Judy is a corporate vice-president with a large multinational corporation:

The thing that I found difficult in my 30s, is when I used to try and figure it all out, I couldn't ever figure out how you could work and have kids. I just didn't see how it was possible. I was working very, very intensely and there were absolutely no role models. In the environment that I worked in, I just couldn't see how you could do it and still have a career. I'm not like a super ambitious person, but I do like working. Then again, I've changed my view on that, and as I've got older I've just become so much more philosophical about life. You know you just figure it out, there isn't any recipe for it; you just figure it out. If you've got a kid, you just figure it out, like everyone else does.

In contrast, for some of us, having children can appear at times to be an attractive and socially acceptable escape route from the pressures of our working life. Janet looks back on her desire for children when she was in her early 30s working as a management consultant:

I suppose I wanted babies, it was as simple as that, a biological need almost. I think it's just time has worn away the desperate urge, and circumstances, I'm just realistic about it. I suppose the times when it was urgent, if I'm really, really honest about it, the times when I was urgent to have children were the times when I was most stressed out at work, and I was seeing them as an escape. I probably wouldn't ever have admitted that at the time, but I would probably have seen it as an escape route.

Wanting the ideal family

As part of our expectations of having it all, many of us wanted children as an essential part of creating the ideal family. Sarah A, who talked earlier about expecting to have children once she had established her career, recalls an incident from her 20s:

When I was 27 I had appendicitis. The ancient old specialist that I went to when I was having my final check made some comment, he said, 'I would advise all women to have their children before they're 25'. I said, 'Well, it's a little bit late for me, why are you advising that?', and he said, 'Oh well, it gets it out of the way, you have actually had them, you've not forgotten, you're at your healthiest and you cope.'

And it's so funny, because at that stage in my life I thought what an old-fashioned attitude, and that's been a quote that's haunted me over the last couple of years, of thinking he was exactly right, I should have just got on with it. I said, 'I haven't met the right person yet', and he said, 'That doesn't really matter' – you know, that really pompous sort, who can say those things. And he got it right, really. I was holding out for the ideal of a total happy family unit, and that isn't really completely necessary.

Fay is 50, and had a strong sense of the sort of family she dreamed of creating:

I wanted a child as part of establishing my family, I think. I'm the youngest of three children and my mother was the youngest of seven children, and you sort of have the feeling that families have their own rhythm in life, they have a pattern that they establish, and whether it's good or bad that's the rhythm that they learn about. I watch other friends' families and see how they do it differently and see the different ways that they establish family. But families are places for me where you may not like each other some of the time but you're part of, and accepted as, a group of people that do things, whether you do them together or apart.

I may have an idealised sense of family, in not having established one of my own, but I just always had this thing about wanting to have my own ... routines, in a sense. I don't mean that in a negative way, but things that you would do around Christmas with your family, you know, like maybe you would establish that you always have stockings at the end of the bed. It's the silly little things that I just thought would be rather wonderful to have – to nurture young people coming up and to get them to look back and think 'That's the way we did it in our family, that's what we had as our way of doing it'.

For many women in established relationships, having a child is the natural next step, and not having children leads to a strong sense that there is 'something missing'. Alice has been married for more than 20 years:

What I'd wanted to do was to create a family, not just a husband and wife unit.

I think there probably came a stage, after a few years of marriage, and I'm not expressing it terribly well, I started to feel that in our lives together as just two people there was something missing. I don't know that I can explain it much better than that. There was something missing, we were very much homed in on each other and each other only, and on our jobs, I suppose, and somehow life was about something rather more than this.

For Caroline, having a family is about creating a sense of belonging:

I suppose it's just that thing to do with family again, isn't it? Love, and I suppose knowing that there's someone you can count on. I really like all my friends, but I sort of feel, if ever there was a crisis, I know that I can rely on my brothers and sisters or my parents. That they will be there. I think it's that whole ... belonging.

A number of women we talked to have suffered from secondary infertility, where they have been able to have one child, but were unable to have any more children, normally for reasons that could not be explained. This is, of course, extremely frustrating and upsetting for all concerned. For these women, not only did having only one child not fulfil their own dreams of having a family, but they also felt terribly guilty about their son or daughter being an only child. Natasha is in her mid-30s, and her son is 6:

One of the biggest driving factors in having another child, as well as fulfilling this idea that I was always going to have two children for me, was for my little boy. As he got older, he asked me constantly why he didn't have a little brother or sister. For me, the greatest sadness is that I haven't been able to give him a sibling.

I found it very, very hard throughout the whole thing, because as he got older, and he was able to articulate what he was feeling, and everyone around him was having babies, he always used to ask me 'Is there a baby in your tummy, mummy?' It was constant. Sometimes, there'd be periods of months when he'd ask me every single day 'When am I going to have a brother or sister, when are you going to have a baby?'

And for Lily, who already has two children from her first marriage, having a child with her second husband was an important part of establishing a 'proper family' with him:

I wanted it for us, I wanted to cement our relationship that this was the love of my life, and I wanted it because I thought it would be good for the children, that it would create a 'proper' family. Instead of two from him and two from me, we'd have something in the middle, that all the kids would love and maybe even have another one, might have twins, I don't know, but I felt it would cement the feeling of family, together. Something to do with the family is crucial. I think it's the clan, I think it's the human need to be part of a unit, and part of the unit is the male and the female and offspring, and that's complete in itself. I can remember my daughter saying to me when she was about 8 [and Lily's first marriage was ending], 'But mummy, we'll never be a mummy and a daddy and two children', and that cut, that hurt.

Wanting to be pregnant and give birth

Another aspect of wanting a child, expressed by quite a lot of women, is the desire to be pregnant and give birth. Not everyone feels strongly about this – I (Louise) didn't have the desire to give birth, and another childless friend jokes about wishing you could get them in a packet and add water! For those of us who do feel it, this desire may be there all along, although for some it seems to become more important as we get older.

Fay, who talked earlier about the rhythms of family life, really wanted to be pregnant:

However much friends have told me that it's not always a good experience, I wanted that experience. It seems to me there's something very basic and primeval about being a woman and being pregnant, and I wanted to have that experience.

Rebecca A, who is in her early 40s, envies the attention and status that pregnant women enjoy:

You know, the way that other women who've been pregnant say 'Oh, how are you feeling, which month are you in now, are you getting the so and so, have you been through such and such?' I wanted that fuss to be made of me. To begin with, it was just the wanting a baby. The wanting to be pregnant, desperately wanting to be pregnant ... I don't know if that's common, and other women like me feel that, but you know, being able to walk around and have this great big pregnant belly that everybody sees, it's like a badge, you know, 'I've done it, I've achieved it'. Proud, and the centre of attention.

When Clare B was 30, her husband stated categorically that he didn't want children. Although she was initially devastated, she quite quickly came to terms with it, and actually felt a sense of relief and freedom at the prospect of life without children. Nevertheless, Clare regrets the fact that she will never be pregnant and give birth, and even considered becoming a surrogate mother:

The biggest regret I think I will have is actually not going through the experience of being pregnant. I think that must be wonderful, and quite extraordinary, to have another person growing inside you. Then obviously giving birth, which perhaps isn't the best time of it from all accounts, but I just think to have felt that must be quite something.

It did go through my mind to become a surrogate mother, and that I could experience pregnancy and childbirth that way, but I just thought 'No, I could end up not giving this child away', and all sorts of things, the problems of actually being a surrogate mother I just thought were too much, I didn't want to have to go through the emotions of giving the child away. I thought I might find that too hard. Actually once you've carried a child and given birth to it, I can imagine you might feel very, very differently, so I decided not to go down that road.

Debbie's husband has children from a previous marriage and did not want any more. For Debbie, the desire was more about breast feeding than actually being pregnant and giving birth:

I'd never particularly wanted to be pregnant, but I'd always wanted to breast feed, I'd really wanted that experience. So there's now no point in having boobs. My first step-grandchild, when he was very small, once rooted for my breast, and I felt very, very strange. That was terribly distressing for me. Everyone laughed, I think his mother laughed and said 'Oh no, there's no milk in there!' and I found that very painful. There was this feeling, there's no point in having breasts, there's no point in having a uterus, there's no point in having periods, there's no point in sex, and I think I felt very alienated from my body. Because I didn't have this strong sense of motherhood in my head, but I just lost my body. There was no point to it.

For Sue, who is in her early 40s, her desire for children is strongly linked to her menstrual cycle:

At this exact point in time, I've reached that emotionally stable point where I'm saying 'They'd be nice but they're not top of my priority list.'

But if you asked me at the end of next week, I'd say 'Absolutely, children are at the top of my priority list', because I'm due to have my period at the end of next week, and I know that I will completely re-evaluate what my priorities are, simply to accommodate that surge of hormones.

I had a bit of a crisis just before my last period. I was away on holiday with my partner, and his kids, and his dogs, and his parents, so this was all right in my face, this happy family, being with a man that I care a lot about. I spent the weekend with about 50 other people, all couples, all with children, screaming, running around, and my hormones were right up there, and I felt like I was going to have a complete breakdown because I just wanted a child. So I know how unstable I can be about it, but my periods of calm are about three weeks of the month.

Rebecca A talked earlier about envying the attention and status that pregnant women enjoy. Here she talks about hormonal problems she is currently experiencing, which mean she is permanently swollen and bloated:

I have this fanciful notion, I'm sure there's nothing medically correct about it at all, but that it's my body's last-ditch attempt to look fruitful and make some man want to make babies with me, because I've got the bust that I always dreamed of having now, and a Titian big belly ... So it really feels that my body's saying 'It's now or never, you stupid woman, don't waste this'.

Jane B is in her early 50s, and has two sons in their late teens, whom she and her husband adopted as babies. Although she thinks the world of her sons, and is fulfilled by them, she still feels sad that one of her basic needs in having children hasn't been fully addressed:

It's still there, it's a ridiculous wish, but it's a huge, huge sadness. A huge sadness, there's absolutely no doubt about it. I wonder whether it is just that feeling of spending nine months being pregnant, thinking about it, and feeling something, being pregnant. I feel it's something that I have never experienced and I just wonder what it would have been like. I don't need, it isn't the baby any more, I don't need that, it is the pregnancy. It's really weird.

Anne B is in her mid 40s:

Now I'm in the position that I have had five miscarriages and the sixth one, I actually carried the baby until it was six months' duration. So it was extremely early when I gave birth to the baby, it was a normal birth, and it lived for a day and then it died. And the feelings that I felt are two-fold: I haven't got a baby, but I've also grieved over a lost baby, because I did have a baby. So I've got mixed emotions, because I haven't got a baby now, but I feel extremely grateful because I did have a baby, even though that baby died. You see, as painful as it is to have lost the baby, there's nothing as marvellous as actually being pregnant, and experiencing being pregnant, a baby growing inside you, and then giving birth to it, even though it wasn't nine months before I gave birth to it, it was only six months, and it died after 24 hours. No one can take that away from me, and that was important.

Wanting to parent

There is no doubt that being a parent is a unique experience, and the desire to parent does seem to get stronger as we get older.

Judy, who talked earlier about her struggles to figure out how to work and have kids at the same time, talks here about how her views on what is important about motherhood have changed:

In the beginning, your priority about having a child is that it has to be your own child, with your own genes, and all the rest of it. Now, I think [the greater prize] is about having another person in your life, a young person, whom you can love and invest in, try and make a difference to their life. I think it's a different type of relationship, it's a unique human relationship between mother and child, that isn't the same as between husband and wife, or friends, or colleagues. It's quite profound.

I (Rachel) had so much love, energy and enthusiasm to give my children. I so wanted to be a mum, to submerge myself in what seemed to be such a vital stage in a woman's life, and many of the women we talked to shared their dreams of a child to love, to care for, to nurture and to teach.

Maria is 40 and currently single:

I'm a bit out of step with my peers who've done the husband–baby thing. I don't think it's just the baby thing, I think it's that wanting to belong. It might be a slightly different feeling in someone who doesn't have a partner. If you've got your live-in boyfriend, then you nurture him; if you're feeling particularly motherly, then you do a lot of snuggling him to your bosom, don't you, but you do have that closeness and that tenderness that I think you would imagine you'd have that intimacy with children, which I think is possibly what this is about.

I think it's that monkey thing, that sort of cuddling thing. That appeals to me, the idea of a little monkey around your neck, in a way that it definitely did not when I was in my mid-20s, say. If I had to carry somebody else's kid, I'd be saying 'Oh God, could someone else carry it, oops sorry, her'. I really noticed it. When this first started happening to me, I thought 'Oh, that's really odd, that's not like me, ooh, I had a tender moment with children. Hello?'

For Janet, who talked about seeing children as an escape from the pressures of work, part of her desire for children was about passing her values on to the next generation:

Because I was so feminist in my outlook on work and things, I think I wanted to pass on my lessons of working as a woman in a really tough, masculine environment. There's a strong feminist streak in me that wanted to carry the flame and pass it on. I guess because I'd had that relationship with my mother, the only girl out of four, she and I had been quite close, and I suppose I wanted to continue that. I did want a daughter, in that sense, to fulfil me, and to pass on that opportunity. Nice to see another generation build on my achievements in work, that sort of thing.

For many of the women we talked to, like Eve, it's about reaching a stage in your life where you want or need to give something to someone else, not just your partner:

What made me decide I did want to have a child in my early 30s was when I thought, I thought about myself all the time, and I suddenly thought 'I've got a lot that I want to give to somebody else now'. I had my relationship with my partner, I was putting a lot into that, but I suddenly thought there's something else that I want to give out too, something else. Then I realised, well obviously I think it's a maternal thing, you want to take care of something that's part of you, and bring it up. I think I would have been a good mother.

Rebecca A, who talked earlier about envying the attention and status that pregnant women enjoy, would like a daughter to educate:

I imagine all the things I would do if I had a child – the books I'd read with them, the trips we'd go on to educational places, that's my thing, so I'm constantly inventing ... if I had a daughter, I'd have done this, and I'd do that. In fact, it's not yet the 'I would have done', it's the 'I will'. Which is ridiculous, because there won't be ...

And as we get older, we may become aware of being out of touch with the world of children. Sally, who wanted to replicate her own happy childhood, talks here about what she feels she's missing:

If you don't have children, what I find a bit sad is that I'm not close to what a child's world is, what are they talking about, the words they use, what's in, what's out, the games, the toys, the expressions and the groups, and what goes on at school. When I see my nieces and nephews, I interview them because I'm actually really interested. If you had kids around you, you'd be hearing it all the time; it's not a big deal, but just missing out on that insight into youth culture, the minds of kids. If you didn't have contact with young children at all you'd just be in a completely different world, and actually not knowing that there's this whole culture there.

For me (Rachel), I'd love to have a good reason to remember the names of all the wild flowers that my mother taught me when I was little, to collect conkers, to do handstands in the swimming pool, to eat cheap sweets ... all the things I loved to do as a child.

And, of course, our own particular history and experience, both as children and as adults, can have a huge impact on our wanting to have a child, or to be a parent.

Debi is in her late 40s. When she was in her 20s, she had a son who drowned in a swimming pool before he was 2 years old. She has not been able to have any more children:

When I fell pregnant I wasn't expecting it to happen, but when it did, it was wonderful. I thought, that's what you're there for, basically. It does make you feel that.

I really enjoyed it, it was fun being a mother. It is one of those kinds of feelings that, unless you've actually experienced it ...

I think perhaps for a lot of people who haven't actually gone through that, yes you have a feeling of getting broody and everything, but you can sort of say 'I've made a choice and I don't go down that route'. Whereas I think it's a lot more difficult when you've actually experienced it and gone through it, and then you can't, that's it, you can't have any more children, that's hard.

Rebecca A has talked about her envy of pregnant women, and her desire to educate a daughter. Although her family and friends think that she is single, she has in fact been in a relationship with a married man for the last 16 years, which has inevitably influenced her desire to be a mother:

Having somebody you are entitled to love, I am entitled to love, is a big part of it. Because I'm not entitled to love him. I'm not his woman; publicly, I'm certainly not his woman. But this, nobody could take away from me.

Wanting a stake in the future

The feeling of wanting a stake in the future, or that we're missing out by not having children, also seems to increase with age.

Debi, who talked earlier about her grief at not being able to replicate the experience of mothering that she had with her son, who died at the age of 2, talks here about her feeling of missing out on the future:

The one thing that I think every woman would feel, anybody would feel, which probably gives this urge to be a mother to so many people, is the fact that you do feel as though the chain doesn't go any further, it stops with you. Then you think 'Gosh, well, I won't have any grandchildren, I won't have that sort of rebirth, regeneration around me'. I think that's quite hard to deal with, from a woman's point of view. Basically, you don't have a future, as most people would see a future.

This feeling is often expressed as sadness at not having someone left to remember you, when you die.

Mary is in her late 60s, and celebrated her golden wedding anniversary this year:

I'd like to leave someone behind to remember me. We're very close, my husband's family and I, but we're all going to go together, we're not leaving anybody. We've got the niece and the nephew, I'm sure they'll give us a thought here and there, but I'd have liked to have someone of my own to have left behind. That seems important, for some reason. It's continuity of your life, isn't it? [That somehow your life still goes on] in other people's memories.

The act of making a will can be particularly traumatic. As Debbie says:

Who do you leave your stuff to? I remember breaking down in front of the solicitor, I don't think she knew what had hit her. That was my biggest thing, 'Who can I leave my things to?' The thing I focused on,

I have a little collection of eggs, ceramic eggs, wooden eggs, I've got one that's a little wooden egg covered in lapis lazuli and inside there's dominos – who am I going to leave my eggs to? It's where does this legacy go?

Wanting your family line to continue into the future can be particularly important for women who have lost their parents early in life. Elizabeth, now in her late 30s, had to have a hysterectomy when she was 20, by which time both her parents had died of cancer:

It's also terribly emotive for me, both my parents being dead, it was a big family line issue. I think it has to be something about the fact that you believe that your own family line has certain strengths and qualities to it that mean that it should be perpetuated. Human beings are quite – I don't know whether selfish is the right word, maybe a little bit arrogant, or whatever. We are all a bit selfish, I think, actually having children to some extent it's about having something in your own image. I think that's what it is, and also this thing of feeling that your time on earth hasn't been totally useless, that you've left something behind, a legacy, it's quite primeval really, isn't it?

The idea of children being the legacy that you leave behind can be particularly important in some cultures. Natasha, who has a son aged 6, would dearly have loved another child:

I believe that children are what you leave behind, sort of thing, they're your legacy, in a way. That really, they are the only thing you leave behind, apart from memories that other people have of you, your children are what hopefully will be what carries on your genes throughout time. It's about time and carrying on the line and family ... family's really important. Also, because I grew up in a very close, Jewish family, very much family orientated, everything was around the family.

Anne B talked earlier about how important it was to her, after five miscarriages, to have been pregnant and given birth, even though her son lived for less than 24 hours:

The other really important thing is, when I was really pregnant, when I got past that stage and I was four months, five months, I don't know when it was that I felt that I was really pregnant, I realised that that's what life was all about. Life. What we're here for is to have children, to pass yourself on and what you have to offer to your children, to then take it forward when you die, you are then going to be taken on to the next generation.

That's when I realised, and I'd not thought that before. That's what life was all about. That's what we're really here for. Because you can often think, you could have gone out a couple of nights ago to this fantastic do, and had the most wonderful time, but does it really matter if you went there or not? What you'd miss, whether you'd done it or you hadn't. What does it really matter, anyway? But actually passing yourself on to your children is just a wonderful, wonderful thing. And I thought that's what life's all about, I realise now what we're here for, and that's to do that.

I think that affected the way I felt afterwards, as well, because that's what I'd felt. Yes, [it made it harder], because you then put everything in its place, what does it mean, exactly, what does it mean, not having children? And it means that, when we die, we die. Whereas if you're a mother, when you die your child then lives on to the next generation, and will then hopefully have children and on and on and on.

Other aspects of the dream

There are other aspects of the dream of wanting a child that defi-nitely seem to intensify with age. Finding a partner, and wanting that partner's child, even when it hasn't been a particularly big issue up to that point, is a major trigger. As soon as Douglas and I (Rachel) became an item, I started to fantasise about which bits of us would turn out to be the dominant genes. I hoped our children would have my cheekbones and Douglas's sense of fun; that they'd be bright, chatty, go-for-it types like we are.

Specific events may trigger our latent desire for children. For Elizabeth, who talked about her desire to perpetuate her family line, it was the pregnancy of close friends when she was in her early 30s, having had a hysterectomy ten years earlier.

I remember one evening when we went out with some really good friends of ours. They were really good time friends, we did lots of socialising with them, lots of drinking with them, we had a really good social relationship with them, and they announced they were pregnant. That was like someone had dropped a boulder on me, for me that was like a realisation suddenly of what I was missing out on. I don't know why it was that moment. I came home, and I remember my husband and I both cried, for what we felt we were missing out on. I suppose that was the moment then that we really started to think about it.

For Marti, the trigger came when she was in her late 30s, and she got to know her brother's daughter:

The first time I felt any connection with a child was when I met my niece, and she looked like me, and I thought this is different. So then I thought 'OK, this is interesting, this is different, this is a different sort of child to the others that I've been used to'. I definitely felt a bond. I definitely felt that she was a family member, and therefore different. So I guess that was a sort of trigger to get me thinking about it.

And many women have talked about feeling increasingly excluded as they get older, and of wanting children in order to be normal, to be like everybody else.

Lara talked earlier about being seen as the homemaker in her family, and being expected to have the 2.2 children. Here, she talks about getting married when she was in her late 30s:

I met this person, who I married six months later, which was completely nuts. I wanted to be normal, I was desperate, really – not to get married, but to get married and have my baby. I know that was really the point, rather than who it was, actually, because I'd had a long affair, and the person I was in love with, whose baby I would have loved to have had, I couldn't have. So I think why I'm stuttering over all of this, is the awareness that not only was I not going to be able to get pregnant, it was too late when the relationship ended, but I lost the relationship, I lost my job and I lost the opportunity to have a baby, literally, all in the space of no time.

Lucy A feels that she has missed out on a huge chunk of normal family life by not being able to have children:

When friends' or family's children, they'll have their 18th, their 21st, university graduation, they'll get married, they'll have children, lots of grandchildren ... you cut yourself off, by not having children, it's forced upon you that you'll miss out on what is a huge chunk of what is a normal family life, and it doesn't just stop by you not having your own children, it goes through generations.

You can go to all these amazing places, but you're still going to see happy families with their children wherever you go, and you're still going to think 'That's what I really, really want'. You know I don't want to get on a plane and go here there and everywhere, I just want to be at home in the garden, have a little child, have a happy family and be 'normal', as we're all led to believe it's 'normal' to have a family.

And as we start to face up to the reality that the child we have dreamed of may not materialise, the desire for a child can become all-consuming. Jane B, who talked about how adopting children failed to fully address her basic need to be a mother, and to give birth, talks here about the time she was trying to get pregnant, before her husband's infertility was diagnosed:

By that time it was all-consuming. If anyone got pregnant I'd be able to smile and be nice, but I'd get into the car and come home and weep, brokenly, I mean it was absolutely ghastly. Then I actually got to the stage where I really felt very, very depressed and felt almost suicidal over it. I kept thinking 'Well, if I had an accident then I wouldn't have to go on', because it became completely obsessive.

CHAPTER 2

Wanting a child – the reality

However long we have dreamed of having children, however detailed and all-consuming our dreams may have been, at some point many of us will have to face up to the fact that our dreams may not come true.

Moments of crisis

For some of us, like Anne A, our dreams may be brought to an abrupt end, in a moment of crisis:

When I was 18, I hadn't seen a period. So my mother took me to see the doctor, who examined me, then I went for tests at the hospital. You can imagine, in 1960, they were very abrupt and just sort of said, 'I'm very sorry to tell you that you won't be able to carry children'. My birthing organs are not properly formed. I had this thing called Turner's syndrome, which unfortunately does go with that. I was devastated. You can imagine, at 18, being told 'Well, you'll never have children'. I was absolutely devastated. My mother was very matter of fact, she's dead now, bless her, but she said 'Oh well, you just get on with it', that was my mother. She said 'Oh well, some people don't want children anyway'. I think she was trying to make me feel better, but it didn't work.

Lucy A married her second husband when she was in her mid-30s. They desperately wanted to start a family and, when it didn't happen, they decided not to hang around but to go straight into IVF. The pre-treatment checks identified that Lucy had cancer:

So instead of having IVF, I was now having a hysterectomy. I felt completely devastated. I could see why the nurse was there, because however strong you think you are, the strongest person in the world, it hits you as though somebody has just put a brick between your eyes, because you just cannot believe it. It's really strange, you're thinking that this news, this information you're being given would just float over you, but it doesn't, it goes straight through into the subconscious, which takes over, and it shocked me how I reacted. I didn't react consciously, it was just the subconscious took over, I had to pretty well pass out, well not pass out completely, but had I been standing I probably would have fallen to the ground.

For a number of the women we talked to, it was the start of the menopause, particularly where this was early or unexpected, that brought their dreams of having a child to an abrupt end.

When Heather was in her mid to late 30s, she was in a relationship and although they had never discussed having children, she decided that if she got pregnant, that would be absolutely fine:

Time passed and I didn't get pregnant and then I was 38, 39, just coming up 40 and I got quite upset about it. I hadn't been feeling very well, quite depressed which isn't me, feeling just generally physically not well at all. I went to my gynaecologist who said 'I'm just going to do some tests', and I thought 'Ooh, maybe I'm pregnant', and it was the menopause, which came as a complete bolt out of the blue.

I have to say, my gynaecologist was wonderful, I remember him saying to me as I sat there with tears streaming down my face, he said 'The trouble is you've had two shocks: one is your body isn't ready for it but it's happening, so somehow physically you've got to be able to accommodate it', and he said 'Psychologically you're not ready for it, so you've got to give yourself time'. He spent a long time with me just talking it through. But there's nothing you can do about it. Once it's there, it's there.

For Clare C, the moment of crisis came when her husband said that he didn't want to do another cycle of IVF:

My husband said he didn't want to do it a second time, because it was so stressful. For him, really, he found it very, very stressful and he didn't like it because it was so unnatural. He hadn't been that keen, but he did it for me, and he didn't want to do it again. When he said that, I couldn't believe it. Absolutely couldn't believe it. I have periodically been angry over the years since, which is now about nine years, when I think about that. But then again, he found it awful. He just couldn't face going through that again.

Agonising decisions

Not all of our dreams end in a single moment of crisis. Many of the women we spoke to wanted a child, but not at any cost, and remaining childless ultimately involved an agonising decision.

Should I stay or should I go? In the space of a few seconds, the time it took for me (Rachel) to hear my husband's 'No children' declaration, I switched from confident, adoring wife to gibbering wreck. How could the man I loved arrive at such an unnatural decision? Was he fatally flawed? Did I still love him … could I still love him … should I still love him? As I described in the introduction, this was my crisis point and a moment of deepest despair.

It took me nearly three months of agonising indecision to finally decide to stay. Three months of looking at all the pros and cons, conducting countless cost-benefit analyses of our relationship, weighing up what I put in and what I got out of loving and living with Douglas. I'd spend an hour, a day, sometimes longer, mentally living with the 'I'm leaving' scenario, examining how the decision sat with me. At other times, I'd live with 'I'm staying', and see how that felt. I considered the question from every angle, in every mood, in different settings, at different times of the day. It was the biggest decision of my life, with no possibility of compromise, no middle way. Whichever way the decision went, it would change the path of my life for ever.

By the end, I felt I knew every facet, every nuance of the issue intimately. I'd lived with it constantly night and day, consciously and unconsciously. I finally came to realise that Douglas's rejection of children was the only aspect of him that I didn't like. It was big, but it was finite and I felt I could accept it. He felt worth the sacrifice.

I've never once doubted my decision, but what I hadn't bargained on was how incredibly hard it would be to live with. It's taken me years, and in some ways I'm still working through the ramifications and probably always will.

Habie and her partner have been trying to have a child for the past seven years, but her partner has now decided not to continue with fertility treatment, leaving Habie with an agonising decision about whether to stay with him or not:

One day I came home and I said 'I've seen my future and it has to have children in it, I'm going to have to leave' and he cried his eyes out, and we both said goodbye. It only lasted a night; the next day I said 'Sorry, forget about that, I'm not leaving.' I can't even bear to leave him for a week...

But he does feel terrible. He looks at me and he sees me crying, or he sees me looking through magazines at babies, and it breaks his heart. He's been convulsed with sobs of guilt, how could he do this to me, but he has to be true to himself. He says 'For five years, I let myself follow your dream. The last year, it was just for you. And I thought, OK, well I'll love this baby when it comes, I'll be a dad, but I wish I didn't have to.' And now he's saying 'Well, I can't subsume myself into you any more than I have in those five years.' But he's losing respect for me because I lost respect for myself.

And for many women, the decision on whether to stay with a partner who doesn't want children is made more complicated by age – if we are already in our late 30s or early 40s, we have to be realistic about our chances of meeting someone else who also wants children, building a relationship with them and our being able to successfully conceive and give birth, all within the small window of opportunity that we have left.

For a number of women we spoke to who are with partners who don't want children, the idea of having an 'accident' has inevitably occurred. Like me (Rachel), they all came to the conclusion that it would be unfair – both to their partner and to the child – and simply wrong. But it's not an easy decision, when we all know women who have taken a different view.

Lucy B had to have both ovaries removed when she was in her early 30s, just six weeks after her wedding. For Lucy, the agonising decision was whether she should pursue egg donation:

I was 33 by that stage, and they say you need eggs of someone under 35 to have the best chance. If I was going to have to recruit an egg donor from among my friends, I had to get my skates on. The difficulty of doing that, I felt I was being very much rushed into making a decision about it. My husband had reservations. I swung from being 'Yes, we've got to do this', anything to have a child sort of mentality, to thinking about the minutiae of all that this meant, the moral, ethical considerations, and the social and psychological impact it could have on the child. So I had two great conflicting things, the force of the biological clock, and my cautious personality.

We went and made enquiries about egg donation, and we had various tests. The consultant we saw there restored my faith in the medical profession, in that he was the first person to show me empathy, and he said 'Gosh, that must have been such a dreadful shock, so soon after you'd got married, when you were setting out in that way.' He said 'There is no rush for you, you've got a healthy uterus, and it's the age of the eggs, the eggs aren't coming from you, you can be 40 and have a 21-year-old's eggs and have a good chance of success.' So that was very positive for me, it seemed to take the time pressure off me and allowed me to explore in counselling what I really thought about the egg donation issue. Ultimately, I decided there were too many ethical dilemmas for me to go ahead with it.

A final area where agonising decisions have to be taken is whether or not to become a single mother, which for some was linked to the decision on whether or not to have an abortion.

Although her family and friends think that Rebecca A is single, for the last 16 years she has been in a relationship with a married man:

Three-and-a-half years ago I discovered I was pregnant, complete accident, certainly not intended at all, and I was over the moon, I just couldn't believe it.

Eventually, when I had it confirmed at the doctor's, I broke the news to my lover and all hell was let loose. Nothing could ever have prepared me for his reaction, which wasn't just 'Oh my God, I don't know what I'm going to do', it was 'You can't have this child; you are not going to have this child.' That really was his mantra for two weeks until I gave in and had an abortion.

I couldn't stand the bullying. He would be here when I got home from work, he'd be here when I got up to go to work, he had keys to the house so he'd be here whenever it was that I was here, he would appear and he would just go on and on and on about what you're planning to do will screw up the lives of my children, they're the ones who matter, you will ruin their lives, this is nothing but a lump of jelly, you can't do this. Then it was, if you do this, I will disappear off the face of the earth, my family won't know where I am, they won't even know if I'm still alive and they'll come on to your doorstep because you'll have ruined their lives. And it was this sort of stuff.

So I gave in. It had never occurred to me that he would do that to me. I was shocked beyond belief. That's partly why I gave in; it was like pulling the rug out under my feet, I had never expected him to treat me that way, to behave so dishonourably. The language he used to me, and the anger he directed at me was such a shock, that didn't help me to be strong.

I phoned the abortion clinic the next day and said 'I'm giving in. This is the wrong thing to do, and I don't want to do this, but I'm giving in. I have no strength left to fight.' At the clinic, there were protesters outside; it's in a neat little residential area, and there were protesters outside telling me, ha-ha, what I was doing was wrong, not telling him, and I screamed my head off, in just hysteria, again, and still even that didn't put him off. I was begging him, 'Don't make me do this', and still he took me in there.

When I (Louise) got pregnant in my mid-30s, as the result of one night with an old flame, I knew that this might well be my last chance to have a child. But, after many, many hours of talking it through with all my close friends, I decided to have an abortion – I just didn't feel that I could cope, emotionally, with being a single mum. Although even then, I could only go through with it by telling myself that it really wasn't too late – I still had time to find a partner and have a child, and that would now be my highest priority. Of course, I didn't do it, and I now recognise that this fantasy was necessary to protect me from the finality of my decision, until I was able to accept it.

Although the decision may have been agonising, the fact that it was a conscious decision has in some ways made my situation easier to cope with. I could have had a child; I chose not to; I know that, faced with the same set of circumstances, I would make the same decision again.

Gradually dawning realisation

For many women, rather than a moment of crisis, or an agonising decision, it has been a gradually dawning realisation that they've left their dream of having children too late, and it's not going to happen.

For Lesley, having children was always something for the future:

Then it suddenly dawned on me that I was about 41 and the children that I'd always been going to have in the next couple of years or so, if ever I really wanted them, time was beginning to run out. And that was just so frightening, because what had I done with that great chunk of years? About 20 years of my life had gone past where actually I'd had quite a lot of good times, I'd had some interesting jobs, all the rest of it, but because of the increasing drinking and all the addictive stuff, it was just like my life had gone past, and it's just such a loss, wasted time. I find myself wanting to cry, even talking about it.

Judy has spent a lot of time reflecting on her childlessness:

I wanted to understand why I got into this position. One of regret and a feeling that I didn't understand what was really most important in my life. I allowed myself to subjugate my expectations as a woman in order to just deal with the reality around me. I didn't realise I was doing it, so I used to think about it a lot but I never realised what corner I was placing myself into, that it was going to become an increasing non-option. I think had I really realised that it was an increasing non-option then I would have dealt with it in a much more dramatic way.

So I worry, I worry well what's it going to be like when you're 60? Because now you look back on it at 50, well 47, and you think 'God I wish I'd known all this when I was 37', and you'd be happy to wind back the clock. So what are you going to think about when you're 60, and you look back to when you were 47, and you say 'God it was still within my power, it was still just within my power and I didn't do it'. So I feel burdened by the whole thing, and the consequences of different routes, and I still get really, really, really frustrated, which is that most people, they just get pregnant. Then you don't have to deal with any of this. You don't have to go on courses, you don't have to have social workers, you don't have to have medical treatment, you just do it.

If I found myself pregnant tomorrow, I would be the happiest person on the planet, because it would just happen, which is how it's supposed to happen. You don't make all these decisions and have to do all these unnatural acts, so I keep saying to myself 'It's no wonder you're traumatised by the whole thing because it shouldn't be like that, it should be (pop), there's a baby, that how is it for 95 per cent of people.' Honestly, if I was pregnant tomorrow I know I would sort everything out. I'd figure out the work, I'd figure out the house, I'd figure out our financial situation, I'd figure out everything – it's just a set of decisions you've got to make.

Janet married for the first time in her mid-20s, and divorced in her early 30s. She was then in a long-term relationship through most of her 30s, but her partner already had children from his previous marriage and didn't want another child. She married her second husband when she was in her early 40s:

With my first husband, I was young, and everybody was having babies all around me, not all, but some of my contemporaries were having kids and it seemed about the right time to do it. With my next partner, it was actually that I really wanted to co-parent with him, because he was such a good father. He is such a nice man, he really is, I suppose I had this idyllic view of what it would be like to bring up a child with him, and I really wanted to do that. With my second husband, he's never been that keen on having kids. Basically we got married when I was 40, 41, something like that. By then, I think, the urgency had died in me a little bit and I guess the reason we're childless is I haven't felt urgently enough about it.

So that's sort of the net position. I've gone through periods of wanting desperately, and now come to the fairly comfortable realisation that having kids in your 40s, when you've just managed to open up your life to 'fulfilling me' as opposed to fulfilling all sorts of other people's needs of me, paying off the mortgage and all sorts of other things, it now became less of an issue, and something I could let go.

Not wanting to give up hope

Even when, deep down, we know that our dream of having a child is just not going to be realised, it can be very difficult to finally give up all hope.

Linda's only daughter was born when she was 29. Linda desperately wanted more children, but when she had not conceived after several more years of trying, tests identified that her husband's sperm was very low in motility, and she was unlikely to conceive again. Despite this, she went on hoping, right up to the menopause:

You're waiting to see every month, of course, if you've conceived, so there's always that, for the next two weeks, you're waiting for your period. Every time your period comes you get so depressed, I can't tell you, it's just this sort of devastating thing. Every month, and you don't get over it. You don't ever get to a point where you can say ... well, of course, when your periods stop, then you do. But until then, you always hope, every month, that you won't get a period. And it's a crushing blow, every single month. So you go into a frump.

So it's this thing hanging over you the entire time. I think that's what gets to you afterwards, it's that you can't let go, you can't. Because you're reminded every month, you can't let go of it, you can't, like with other things, say 'OK I'm going to put that one to rest', because every month you have this bloody reminder.

A number of women we spoke to admitted, rather guiltily, to secretly hoping that they were pregnant each time their period was a few days late, even when rationally they knew that they were going through the menopause, and felt that they had (or should have) accepted that getting pregnant just wasn't going to happen for them.

Penny B is in her late 40s, and gave up trying to conceive through IVF almost ten years ago:

Even after IVF, I was having periods and I used to think, when I didn't have one, I'd think 'Maybe I'm pregnant'. I used to live in this hope all the time. Secret as well, because as far as my husband was concerned, we'd moved on. We'd done this moving on bit. So it almost felt like, again, a failure, an admission of failure, to admit that actually I'm still harbouring secret hopes that I might be pregnant, because it was sort of revisiting, going back again.

That's one of the hard things, I think, it's not a continuum like that, you go sort of backwards and forwards. So although you're moving along, you're sort of zig-zagging backwards and forwards all the time. Whereas men say, 'You're moving on, why haven't you moved on to here?', we're sort of fluttering around. Sometimes you do hurtle forwards and then hurtle back again.

We are particularly grateful to Debi, who sent us the following email a few days after talking to us for the book, which illustrates so poignantly the internal struggle between hope and reality:

> *Dear Rachel,*
> *I am sitting here now and thinking, I am thinking the thoughts that so many of your future readers will have felt, will feel or will be feeling, so I am relaying them to you.*
> *I am thinking that I am 47 years old, I know that I am going through the menopause but my period is late … so where does that leave me …. It leaves me again with hope of the one thing I have always wanted, another chance. I know that I am going through a divorce but am still prepared to think that the result of a brief liaison, when I was still menstruating, may just result in pregnancy (who am I kidding?). I am also thinking that there may be a chance that more could develop from this friendship but nevertheless to pronounce myself pregnant would be an awful thing to do to someone just out of one relationship and with three children to support. What would his reaction be, he is a very decent fellow and we had already agreed that this would be something that both of us could enjoy with no strings. You see, a few days late and the thoughts that well up in ones head are amazing. The more you are late, the stronger the thoughts become, the more hope wells up inside. I know I would support myself financially (here I go again) so that isn't a problem, I read more into my horoscopes than I should and I feel pathetic for doing so. In the back of my mind I know that within a couple of days I will start my period – and even worse just before I get to that stage I will find myself asking for a pregnancy test. Is it possible to will the colour on the swatch? No. Will I buy a pack of two just in case? Yes. just for a few moments, hours, days a feeling grows inside, the stomach swells up (it always does, doesn't it, just before a period) and you find yourself touching your stomach and floating off to a dream world.*
> *At the end, after so long, there isn't really a disappointment, it's just an acceptance and now I don't take it badly ….*

But those hours are enjoyable, those moments of expectation, followed by those moments when you briefly question your God and your feelings. Momentary selfish thoughts. These are very private thoughts, but so real and so painful for just a few brief moments, then they are forgotten until the next time. The next time when all those other times come back to you and you yoyo between what you know is realistic and what you want to believe.

Rachel, I felt I should really pour these thoughts out as I feel them. No doubt tomorrow I will be back again to my prag- matic self, in fact I am already almost there, indeed I am almost willing myself to start my period so I can stop such stupid thoughts.

Just thought an insight as it happens might help you for the book.

Good luck and hope to see you again sometime.
Debi

P.S. I am going to send this really fast before I feel stupid so if it seems like a load of rambling rubbish please ignore.

There are a number of ways in which we fuel our dreams, keeping hope alive against all the odds. Looking at our family history is one way that was talked about by a number of women. Habie, who talked about the agonising decision of whether to stay with her partner or leave him, talks here about her family history.

The fact that my mother had six children and the last one was born when she was 44, gave me this completely false role model that all women could have babies well into their 40s, and there's nothing wrong with that, it happens, and that's fine. There's no miscarriage in our family, no aunts, no grandparents, no cancer, no nothing. I just assumed that I came from a breeding family, and that therefore when I wanted to have my children I would.

Habie also goes on to talk about the possibility of overseas adoption, which again was mentioned by a number of women we talked to:

I think most women who want children know that in China, to adopt a baby girl, the age limit is about 52, so there's a fair whack of time where, in a previous generation, you'd have thought you're in your 40s, you're finished. Now we know you can both have babies naturally, you can give birth in your 40s, and you can adopt in your 40s, at least abroad. So it is possible.

Hilary Mantel, in her autobiography *Giving Up the Ghost*, writes:

> *Children are never simply themselves, co-extensive with their own bodies, becoming alive to us when they turn in the womb, or with their first unaided breath. Their lives start long before birth, long before conception, and if they are aborted or miscarried or simply fail to materialise at all, they become ghosts within our lives. [...] In a sly state of half-becoming, they lurk in the shadowland of chances missed.*

Linda talked earlier about waiting every month to see if you've conceived, never really getting over it. Here, she talks about her sense that she has other children, whom she has never met:

I did think that somehow there were these phantom children, and I can't really explain it, but that there were. I did have children somewhere, somehow, or would have, that just never materialised. I've had a very good life, I've been lucky … but it doesn't take away from that pit feeling, of knowing there's more there. Knowing that there are these other children, it's very hard to explain, that there are other children in me, that I want to know. You know they're there, and you want to know who they are. Maybe it's just plain curiosity. It's almost like … I read about missing limbs, I think, that's something like the feeling, this phantom limb thing.

Linda's conviction touched something in me (Rachel). I think the fact we're born with all our eggs led me to feel I had children-in-waiting, that they existed, if only in my mind's eye, tantalisingly real and yet, at the same time, utterly elusive.

And I (Louise) could really identify with Marilyn, who is in her early 50s, when she talks about the impact of other people's pregnancies, particularly as reported in the media:

I find it very difficult not having children. Every time I see the newspaper and they say there's somebody of 53 or 62 has had children, I think 'Oh well', and my heart lifts.

Putting your life on hold

While there is still hope of fulfilling the dream of having a child, it can be hard to avoid putting other aspects of your life on hold.

A number of women talked about taking decisions, or indeed failing to take decisions, about their working lives because they were planning or assuming that they would be having a baby in the near future. Here are three of them:

I think career-wise, I never did anything because I thought I'm going to get married. Once we got married I didn't do anything, because I thought we would have children. Then we started trying after a year or two, and actually it was on our 10th wedding anniversary that our daughter's adoption was finalised. But I didn't really think about it, it was just assumed. (Caroline, who met her husband when she was just 19)

When I left my first job, I could have completely retrained and become a teacher, and the government would have given me funding, or I could just do a refresher course in secretarial. Because in my head I was going to get pregnant and have a family, I just chose to do the secretarial course. A big mistake. (Jane B)

We decided that we'd try for children, and nothing happened. I left my job, which in hindsight was not the greatest of things; I should have stayed on, but in fairness, although I loved the work, I didn't like the people I was working with, so it was kind of an added impetus to leave. And I honestly thought my life was going to be going in a different direction. I left with a view to establishing myself as a freelance person, that people were used to dealing with at home, and then could sort of slot in the childcare with that. Nothing happened. (Clare A)

Habie, who talked earlier about her family history, and the possibility of adopting a child from overseas, is currently very stuck, with many aspects of her life on hold. She is unwilling to give up her dreams of having a child, but at the same time finds it almost impossible to do anything else in her life:

So it is completely, it's colouring my life; it's covering everything with a veil. But it's actually possibly destroying it. Come back in five years' time if you do a follow up to your book, and see if I was one of the one's who made it or who didn't. It could kill me, you know. It could absolutely kill me, because if it destroyed my relationship and I went into a spiral of solitude and loneliness and not able to work, and then not having any money, and having to live on my own in a one-bedroom flat, with no kids and no man and no nothing ... all of that because of the childlessness, that could happen. It could kill me, I don't know. I always wanted to have the identity of a creative person, but I realised in the last five years that my creativity was to be a mother, and not having it has left me feeling like nothing.

And Wendy, who is a nutritionist, talks here about the impact on some of her clients (and herself) of desperately trying unsuccessfully for a second child:

Sometimes they can be so busy on this route to get the second child that they're not even enjoying the childhood of the first, it's a kind of irony. To a certain extent I've been there myself, rushing off in the middle of the night to do IVF treatments and leaving my daughter, I mean it's crazy.

Moments of truth

Even when we think we've learned to live with the reality of our childlessness, there can still be times when we have to face up to it all over again. Clare A, who had given up her job and gone freelance in anticipation of having children, talks about a 'blip' she had when she reached 40:

I started thinking about all this again, because obviously lots of people do manage to have children into their 40s. Then I started having fairly bad gynaecological problems, I'm not quite sure what they were, but I had very heavy bleeding. So I basically had gynaecological problems, thoughts about being 40, thoughts about never having had children, so it was all quite hard to deal with.

Obviously, I'm eight years on from there now, and I find it more upsetting thinking back to how I was, than I do now. OK, I sit here, crying about it now, and occasionally feel quite, you know, a pang when I see other people's children, or hear other people talking about family undertakings.

Clearly the menopause is a significant milestone for all women, but particularly so for those of us who are childless, but not through choice. When we started working on this book, I (Louise) was 44, and hadn't given any thought to the menopause – it was far in the future, surely? Then, at the end of last year, I was chatting to my doctor, and idly speculating about how I would know whether I was menopausal, given that I have a type of coil fitted that means that I don't have periods. We needed to do a blood test for something else, so my doctor requested an FSH (follicle stimulating hormone) reading.

The results came back, showing that I was clearly not just menopausal, but post-menopausal – I had been through the menopause without even realising it! My initial reaction was surprise and shock, and then my rational mind took over, telling me that this was in fact good news; I didn't have to worry about all those ghastly symptoms that I'd started to hear other, older women talking about.

But when I got back from my trip to the supermarket later that day, having bought a box of mince pies (not something that normally forms part of my diet) and eaten them all at one sitting, I realised that perhaps I wasn't feeling quite so happy about the news. Over the next few days, I talked to various friends about it, including Rachel and another friend who is a family doctor, and I now really do see the benefits of where I am. But it surprised me, thinking I was quite OK with my childlessness now, how much the news affected me, without really realising it.

Lesley is 50, and talked earlier about how, for her, having children was always two or three years in the future:

I think I probably accepted emotionally fairly well about five years ago that it was pretty bloody unlikely that I'd ever have kids. Yes, I've got some regrets, but the reality is I've got a nice life and actually, no, now is not the time.

But it's one thing to accept that, it's quite another thing to have your body start to pack up on you and tell you 'Well, you can't'. That is, it's all very well to have free choice, I guess, it's quite another thing to find that even if you wanted to, you can't. Almost a sort of cheat ... it's like I spent all those years, having whatever form of birth control, and on occasions being terrified that I was pregnant, and suddenly to find that actually, well, it's not going to happen anyway, it's a bit like the whole cosmic joke of being 50 in the first place. Because mentally, emotionally, I feel like about 17, and it doesn't seem real. It just seems like 'Hey, God, you're playing a funny one here, how did this happen?'

It's a real split and a conflict, it's like I've just about got to the stage where it's not going to happen, and that I think is just about OK by me, but what do you mean you're telling me I can't anyway? It's like being a little child, and wanting what you can't have. Actually, while I've got the choice, I'll choose not to, but if you tell me that I haven't got the choice then I'll get angry about it. The grass is greener syndrome.

For Shirley, who is 70, and has been widowed for 20 years, the moment of truth was the realisation that her marriage had probably never been consummated:

Nobody really spoke to me about sex. Only a few years ago, I was talking to a girl, and she said that she had been to the doctor after she was married and it hadn't been penetrative. And so I suddenly thought, 'Oh, do you think that happened to me?' And I was terribly upset, because it was all in vain, all those years of wanting and hoping, every month, every month, and people would be saying nasty remarks to me and I couldn't say anything. Just every month, all the time, hoping, it was agony, really, that was.

For many women, there are certain times of the year that are more difficult than others. For Sally, as for a number of the women we talked to, Christmas is particularly difficult:

I don't really like Christmas any more, I used to love Christmas, and I feel sad about that. Christmas is a bad time, because it is a lot about the joy that children get from Christmas, and nativity plays, and Father Christmas, and the fun and the games that you might play and things like that. You join in with other parts of your family, but it's such a shame. I don't mind it too much now, it's OK, but there was a time where I just thought I can't go through Christmas and I seriously was considering volunteering at Crisis, I thought I'll really do something different, I just don't want to do this, it will be absolutely awful.

Now, what we tend to do is sweep up the elderly relatives, thinking 'Well we've made their Christmas nice', and then go off somewhere. These other friends of ours go off sailing in the Bahamas, or Christmas in New York or something like that. Of course, if you don't have those ties, you're not going to have a conventional Christmas, so you have a completely unconventional one, and turn your back on it.

For Elisabeth it's Mothering Sunday that is particularly difficult to cope with, as it reinforces not only her own childlessness, but also the loss of her mother when she was only 16.

And for Lara, who is in her mid-50s, it's holidays:

That's when it hits me most, holidays for me are the most difficult, because even if I go with a group of people, you know, when it gets to my age, people are always talking about their children, and if they're not talking about their children, they're talking about their grandchildren. So you again feel the odd one out. You just can't help it, you are. You are the odd one out. It is very, very difficult.

Many women have to deal with issues in their working lives that reinforce their own sense of loss, and that can be particularly difficult. During the research for this book, we've spoken to a midwife, a family doctor and a human resources manager (who has had to counsel staff about unwanted pregnancies), all of whom have really struggled with this, even considering changing career because of it.

Anne B is in her mid-40s, and went through the menopause almost 10 years ago, after having five miscarriages and giving birth to a premature son, who lived for only 24 hours. For Anne, it's taken most of that time to get over the pain of seeing other people's babies:

I can't bear people moaning about their children. 'I've been up all night' or 'I've been awake since 5 o'clock', and moaning about their child. How dare they, because they don't know how lucky they are. I have felt, you know when you go shopping and you see a little baby in a pram, and your heart is just pounding, because you want that baby. You really do. This has gone on ever since. For the first time we were out a couple of weeks ago, and I looked at a little baby and just thought 'Isn't that lovely, isn't that a lovely baby', and it's the first time I've ever been able to do that. It's taken all that time. Funnily enough, I feel I can understand why people take babies now. Not that I would, but I thought I can understand that, which I could never understand before.

In her professional life, Anne is a senior police officer.

CHAPTER 3

The fertility business

As you are reading this book, you may have already been through fertility treatment unsuccessfully. Alternatively, you may be wondering whether some form of fertility treatment would be right for you.

The purpose of this chapter is not to offer a review of the treatments available – this information is readily available elsewhere, and our research suggests that any woman who is seriously considering Assisted Reproduction Techniques (ART) will quickly become a mini expert on the subject!

Instead, what we are aiming to do here is to provide a fuller picture of the process from an emotional perspective. If you have already been through the experience, you can perhaps feel less isolated by hearing of other women's experiences. If, on the other hand, you are considering ART, you will be better informed, can make the decision that is right for you and perhaps be able to manage your own expectations more appropriately if you hear about the experiences of women who have already been through the process.

In order to provide this information from an emotional perspective, we have spoken not only to women who have been through various fertility treatments, unsuccessfully, but also to a number of fertility counsellors.

Considering treatment

For those of us who have no direct experience of fertility treatments, when we think of ART what immediately comes to mind is the constant drip feed of 'miracle baby' stories in newspapers and women's magazines. The more extreme of these – beginning in the 1990s in the US with the case of a woman who gave birth aged 63 and, in Europe, the case of the 62-year-old Italian who gave birth; and, more recently, the 66-year-old Romanian who became the oldest woman ever to give birth in early 2005 – seem to get burnt into childless women's brains, and have been frequently cited by the women we've talked to.

These kinds of stories suggest that any woman entering ART will be able to have a child. And indeed, if a couple have unlimited financial resources, and unlimited physical and emotional resilience then, as one fertility counsellor we spoke to said, almost any woman can indeed have a child. Having that child may involve the use of a donor egg and/or donor sperm, and she may not even carry the child herself, but almost any woman can take delivery of a newborn baby.

The reality, of course, is that the process is incredibly traumatic and demanding. As Alison Bagshawe, Senior Fertility Counsellor at Guy's Hospital in London, told us:

Emotionally, it's like a roller-coaster ride and each treatment cycle is probably more like the Grand National. You've got to have stamina, you've got to have staying power and each hurdle you get over is just one more hurdle and you soon get up to the next hurdle and you have to get over that. You need resilience to cope, and you need support – it can be an endurance test.

And the reality is also that the majority of women trying to have a baby through ART will not succeed. For a moment, let's look at the statistics in terms of failure rates, rather than the success rates that are normally quoted. First, failure rates are very high, and have not reduced significantly over the last ten years – for example, on average, somewhere between 80 and 85 out of every 100 cycles of In Vitro Fertilisation (IVF) will not result in a live birth. Secondly, failure rates vary dramatically with age – for women under 30, they can be as 'low' as 3 out of 4, but for women of 40, they rise to 9 out of 10, and by the age of 45 the failure rate is virtually 100 per cent unless donor eggs are used (Human Fertilisation and Embryology Authority (HFEA) statistics).

If you are considering entering fertility treatment, the fertility counsellors we have spoken to all recommend acknowledging up front that the treatment might fail and trying to view it, however difficult that might be, as a route that you want to explore rather than as a process that guarantees delivery of a baby. Deborah Vowles is a counsellor who has worked on reproductive issues with couples who have life-threatening illnesses, or conditions that might put a baby at risk. As she says:

I always bring up the question: 'What if it doesn't work?' One of my reasons for doing it is that, this is going to cost you a lot of money, it's going to cost you a lot in time, it's going to cost you a lot in emotion, every period counts, your life is going to be governed by this, sex takes on a different meaning, periods take on a different meaning when you start down a fertility journey, do you want to do this?

What I think is important is that you don't get caught up in the glossy brochure, baby purchase thing. The disappointment is going to be there anyway, but playing out the fantasy even further probably makes that disappointment even more. It felt right to me, it felt ethical to me, I think people found it helpful to be pushed a little bit.

For me, it's something about taking responsibility for the decision, rather than putting it 'out there' with others taking control. If you don't get pregnant, it isn't the fertility clinic's fault. It's about trying to be adult about this decision, it involves a whole load of things, let's make it as active a decision as we can, let's make it as adult a decision as we can, let's make it as independent a decision. It's taking ownership – I want to do this, I want to go ahead with this, I'm prepared to take the risks, I'm prepared to take the disappointment. So I think it's the beginning of the grieving process.

And as Liz Scott, Fertility Counsellor at the Assisted Conception Unit of the Lister Hospital says:

The one factor that has been taken away from infertile women is the control over their own fertility, and that's enormous. For so many of us, we've learned from almost primary school age that if we work hard we can achieve. So many people we see are real achievers in their own right, done well in life, found a partner and made a life together, made a home together, and now for the first time, perhaps even as a couple, wanting to achieve something, and there's nothing within their control, as they see it, that's going to change the outcome.

I would encourage folks to be looking at this issue of what brings them in for treatment, what control limits they can put into that particular journey, and how they can have some element of planning around that. One of the issues might be how many treatments they are financially able to have or are prepared to look at in terms of moving forward. I find very often if couples or individuals have done that kind of elementary planning process, then they're often in a better position to look at moving forward.

I then encourage them to look at their coping mechanisms and the skills that they have. All of us, as human beings, have developed really good coping mechanisms and skills by the time we have reached the age that most women are when they come into treatment, but very often when they're so thrown, it's like they just lose sight of it at that period of time. So I encourage them to recognise that. How can they recapture some element of control? Even if it's something as elementary as when they might choose to come in for the next treatment.

Concerns about treatment

A number of women we spoke to had concerns about ART. Helen's husband had a vasectomy before he met her, after having two children in his previous marriage. They have talked many, many times about whether he should have the vasectomy reversed:

So we did talk about whether we would do the roulette wheel, you know kind of let's have it done, let's see whether it works, let's see whether I get pregnant. We also talked about, and it's back to the rational piece of me again, I suppose, what would happen if we did take that decision, to have the vasectomy reversed – which to me was a bit like jumping off a cliff – and it wasn't successful, then what would we do about that? Would we then go into the next step, you'd normally be looking at IVF, and I'm personally opposed to IVF, because for me every embryo is a child, and you have to fertilise X embryos, and so many of them don't get used etc., so for moral reasons I didn't want to go down that route, I wasn't comfortable with that at all.

I think my concern was that if we take this, to me what is a kind of a watershed decision, to have the vasectomy reversed, then we'd be getting ourselves geared up to really wanting children. I think you then set the expectation, or the anticipation, that you really, really want them, and when it doesn't work, your disappointment factor is absolutely huge.

Helen has moral concerns about IVF and another one of the women we spoke to, Hira, has not been able to have the only fertility treatment that might help her, because of her religion. Her husband is infertile, but Donor Insemination (DI) is not permitted as they are Muslims.

Jane B really didn't feel that DI would be appropriate for her and her husband, and was also appalled at the way it was proposed by their consultant:

The consultant then suggested that we had DI, and I can remember feeling quite strongly, with my personality, that we actually couldn't do that. Even though I desperately wanted a baby of my own, I felt that it would have to be a shared thing. If we did DI, they were very crass really, they said what they do is they go and do it, you select a donor and everything else, and then you go home and you have sex with your husband and if you get pregnant you pretend that it's his. Well, what a load of rubbish! Who were they trying to kid?

A number of women have expressed their concerns about Intracytoplasmic Sperm Injection (ICSI). Caroline's gynaecologist suggested that she and her husband should try ICSI after three unsuccessful cycles of IVF:

I remember, even now, I didn't think ICSI's a very good idea. I think it's bad enough that you've got the sperm and egg in a dish, as it were, but I think that with ICSI, you don't even know which sperm they're taking, I don't really like that idea. ICSI is when they actually get a single sperm and inject it into the egg to fertilise the egg, rather than just leaving them swimming around, and the best one ... I just remember thinking, but that sperm might be the worst in the bunch, that sperm might have all the genetic faults.

Once you are attending a particular clinic, then in the UK at least, by law you must be offered counselling by that clinic before you consent to treatment. However, if you are at the stage of considering whether ART or a particular treatment is for you, then it can be difficult to find an opportunity to discuss these types of concern with the clinicians. Even if you do, you may or may not meet with a sympathetic response – their focus is likely to be on maximising success rates, and very often the sorts of concerns that have been expressed to us are moral or emotional, rather than simply medical.

Emotional costs

The emotional roller-coaster of trying to conceive with ART can be even greater than the swings of hope and despair experienced when trying to conceive 'naturally'. Fay spent about 5 years in her 30s trying to get pregnant, including one unsuccessful cycle of IVF:

I think the IVF was just like an enhanced devastation of what had been happening on a monthly basis, really, plus you've been through this enormous event of being pumped with hormones and going in for blood tests ... I can't even remember, I think I've blocked a lot of it out because it was very hard.

For Penny, going into IVF treatment meant that she avoided dealing with her grief for a number of years. Penny is now in her late 40s, and her only daughter was born when she was in her mid-30s. Several years later, Penny had an ectopic pregnancy:

I can remember coming round and feeling absolutely wretched. I just cried for a week ... plus. For the loss, because I knew that my other tube was blocked and I knew that was it. This one had ruptured, so that was it. They gave me names of counsellors to go and see and things like that, but I just thought I didn't really need that. I remember I just couldn't stop crying.

I remember seeing a young doctor who came round, and explaining, and he was saying 'Why are you so unhappy?' He said 'But then you're right for IVF, that's what IVF's all about.' I said 'Well, I'm too old', and he said 'No, no, you're exactly right for IVF. You know you can carry a child, it's just your tubes, that's what it's for, IVF.' He said, 'I promise you, you'll have a baby within a few years.' I think in some ways it stopped my grieving process, because then there was this great big hope suddenly that there would be something else. Being sort of right, next project, right I'll get over this grieving bit and then we'll move onto the next one.

The whole process of infertility testing and fertility treatment can be incredibly stressful, and for a significant number of the women we talked to, the stress was increased by insensitive or poor handling by the medical profession, particularly for some of the older women who were having testing or treatment in the 1960s or 1970s. This distress can remain with women for years, or even decades.

Mary is now in her late 60s, and went through testing in the late 1960s:

There was no such thing as infertility clinics, you went to a gynae clinic, saw a gynaecologist, and sat in a waiting room with dozens of other women who were there with fibroids, probably cancer of the uterus, you know, really serious medical problems. And then there was us. Who just wanted a baby. Which was all wrong, wasn't it, it just wasn't right.

I didn't like the consultant, the minute I lay on the bed. She did that, [squeezed my breasts] and I thought 'What's that telling her?', whether it was to see if they were real, then examined me and asked me a few questions. She asked if we had been taking precautions prior to starting trying and I said 'Yes', and she said 'My, my, now we're a sorry little girl, aren't we?' I thought, 'I don't like you very much.'

I went into hospital in the mean time and had this D&C and insuf-flation. We were told the results of that by the sister on the ward who walked around, and in a loud voice at the end of everybody's bed said 'Your tubes are free, you're OK, yours are blocked, doctor's coming to see you, your tubes are free, your tubes are free', this was all around the ward ... it's horrendous, when I look back on it. We just accepted that as the norm, which it was.

Even by the late 1980s, the situation wasn't necessarily much better. Clare A talks about the way her husband's infertility was commu-nicated to them. After the tests had been carried out, Clare and her husband moved house, and never received the results from the hospital:

So somehow in the terrible confusion, we didn't cotton on as quickly as we should have, that there was a problem. We started with a new doctor, and said 'Well, we've had these tests, we don't know what happened.' We got sent to another hospital, and I don't know if they'd somehow accessed the original tests, because we were wheeled into a room and more or less told bluntly, 'Right, that's it, your husband's massively infertile, you'll never get pregnant, it's not even worth looking at you' (to me).

Actually, the words we were told, he looked down at the form, addressed the doctor who was sitting next to him, and said 'Oh yes, Mr so and so, the clearest case of sub something sperm production I've ever seen.' That was how we were told.

Ten years on from her experiences, Anne B is still angry with the medical profession, and upset by the treatment she received:

The medical profession have got this thing, that if you have three miscarriages, then they will then undertake tests. I think that's too much. I think they should do it sooner. Because, right, yes, lots of people have one miscarriage, but two? I think they should think about people's ages, circumstances and things like that, and they shouldn't just be so quick to dismiss it as a normal thing. What they say is, you have three miscarriages, and then they'll start investigations as to why. I think that there is something wrong, if you get to three, if you have two, then there's a problem.

So [after five miscarriages and the death of my premature baby] I went back to this consultant, and he said to me there's nothing wrong with me. I said 'I'm very sorry, but there is. There is something wrong with us. It doesn't take any intelligence to know that there's something wrong. I want to go for further advice, I want a second opinion, I want to see someone who knows what they're doing.' He said 'I assure you, you try again, there's no reason why you shouldn't have a baby.' I said 'I'm sorry, there is something wrong.'

Anne finally got to see her specialist, who was able to determine what the problem was. Sadly, by the time Anne was emotionally ready to consider trying again, her menopause had already started.

We would all like to think that the above examples are history, and that this sort of insensitive treatment wouldn't happen today. Sadly, this isn't the case. In a recent round-up of complaints to the HFEA about licensed fertility clinics, more than 70 per cent of all complaints related to the consultation, information, attitude or response of the clinic to complaints. Complaints included such comments as: patients feeling that the centre was only interested in making money; patients feeling part of a conveyor belt system; and patients feeling that they had been treated like slabs of meat. Indeed, one leading London IVF doctor is apparently known to his patients as 'Captain Insensitive'.

To be fair to the clinicians, it is inevitable that they will be focused more on the medical issues than the emotional ones, but there is no doubt that poor communication or insensitive handling of women's distress can add greatly to the emotional costs of fertility treatment.

Physical costs

Physically, the nature of the fertility treatment process can be gruelling, particularly over multiple treatment cycles. As Alison Bagshawe, of Guy's Hospital in London, says:

Each time you go round, you get more and more exhausted. I'm talking about IVF and probably to a lesser extent some of the other treatments. It really can debilitate people.

Fay, who talked earlier about the enhanced devastation of trying to get pregnant by IVF, describes the process as brutal:

I just got into this routine about blood and vaginal scans, which is something normally you psych yourself up to and you have every now and then, and you accept it because as a woman you know you need certain investigations. But I was having these things so frequently it was almost, it sounds horrible, it was almost go in, sit down, open your legs and let them get on with it.

I think it took me a long while to get over that. I didn't like my body at that stage very much, I didn't like what was being done to it, I didn't like the fact that I was completely out of control, because all the hormones they pump into you meant that I put on a vast amount of weight, and that had always been an issue for me, trying to control my weight, and then afterwards trying to get back into some normal pattern of weight, and get back to a normal physical rhythm, took quite a long time. I just felt that I'd been messed about with, really, in a way that was very intimate. It just felt to me almost like you'd been stripped bare and been completely exposed.

For Clare A, who talked about the way her husband's infertility was communicated, it was the physical effects of the drugs she was given that led her to stop trying DI:

We had a couple of goes and I found the whole thing, I must say, it was minor in comparison with what people go through to do a full IVF, although I did have to take drugs and things, I cannot imagine how people cope with doing many cycles and taking all the drugs. The drugs that I had made me feel completely at sea. So we tried this twice, and in the end I decided that what you were being put through, and in the end it wasn't even going to be your husband's, it just didn't really feel right to continue with that. So we tried twice and then stopped. I just found it totally dehumanising.

Nine years ago, Clare C had a single cycle of IVF, and she talks here about the physical and emotional after-effects:

I'm an emotional person. I've always been an emotional person, but I don't know why it hit me so hard. There are other words involved in grief, like loneliness and despair, and hopelessness, all of which I just touched into. Perhaps, also, because I had various drugs. Women are very emotional around pregnancy anyway, and not only had I been pregnant for a short time and lost the babies, but I also had various drugs pumped into me, progesterone, my body was pregnant, my breasts were very sore for a long time after the babies had gone. It was awful, dreadful. I don't think that's ever left. I still can't believe, when I have a period, how on earth can I keep having these periods and not get pregnant, because I still feel so ready to conceive.

And although complications only happen in a very small percentage of cases, when they do happen, this can be devastating. Natasha is in her mid-30s and talks about her experience of IVF last year:

You basically have a 1 per cent chance of getting this ovarian hyper-stimulation syndrome, which is like a side effect of IVF when your ovaries go into this mad stimulation phase after they take the eggs out. It's only 1 per cent of people. I got that, and I was very, very ill after they took my eggs out, and the whole process was horrible. The drugs and the stress that it puts on you, it's horrible, the way it makes you feel is horrible, the injecting is horrible, the fact that it rules your life for those six weeks, you can't do anything else really, everything revolves around your appointments, your scans ... it takes over your whole life.

I kind of knew it was going to be like that, but what I didn't reckon on was having this complication at the end. So after they took the eggs, we had great success in the laboratory, I had 12 eggs that fertilised with my husband's sperm, so we had 12 embryos waiting to be put back, but then I got really ill, and basically your ovaries are about that big, my stomach was like it was pregnant and I couldn't move, it was like having two cannon balls inside me, it was horrible. I ended up passing out here one day, and being rushed into hospital.

Social costs

As well as the emotional and physical costs of ART, there can also be big social costs. While you are going through treatment, it can be difficult to avoid putting other aspects of life on hold. Sally spent five years trying to get pregnant, including four cycles of IVF:

It's pretty soul destroying, and what's really difficult about that, and I think anybody that's trying for a baby for a long time, whether it's IVF or whatever they go through, it's how you put your life on hold for quite a long time. Because you're waiting to see if this thing happens, so you don't make decisions, you don't sell your house and move somewhere else, or move job, or whatever, you can't because you don't know whether you're going to have a baby, you don't know what your life's going to be. So I look back on that and almost think, gosh, not exactly so much time wasted, but 4, 5, 6 years of my life were waiting to see if this would happen, as opposed to getting on with it.

If it wasn't for that, I think we wouldn't be living where we are, we would have sold the flat and moved, we wouldn't be here. The flat was too small, but we delayed moving, we didn't want to move, we didn't know where, I didn't want to move away from my doctor, I didn't want to start again with someone else, I didn't want to go to a different clinic, you know it was really important to have that support around.

And as Sally's husband, Jock, adds:

For five years, your life is suspended, you can't do things, you can't plan. If you go on holiday, if you're going through a cycle of these things you've got to make sure that you can take the stuff with you. If you're doing anything, even to do with business, meetings, ... sometimes we had to arrange for, I wouldn't do the injections, because I'm scared I'd do something wrong, butterfingers, so we got all the injections done at the clinic, or by arrangement with another clinic whenever Sally was away somewhere. So we had to arrange physical things like this, going on a business trip, to arrange a hotel with a clinic nearby to be able to do it. Or bring in a nurse, or something.

Deciding whether or not to tell people about the treatment can also create additional stress. As Sally goes on to say:

There were quite a lot of unexplained absences, and I suppose I chose to do it that way, I could have chosen to just let everyone know, and some people are very open about I'm going through IVF and all the rest of it, but I didn't want people at work to know because I just wanted to keep it separate, and I didn't want to be the subject of their kind of speculation or gossip or sympathy or anything else, I just didn't want them to know.

I can't remember at what point I told people, mum, obviously, my family, some of my friends, but I can't remember at what point I told them all, but by the end of it they all knew. You had to choose who you would tell if you were going into another IVF attempt and what stage you were at, because if you told a lot of people, then people would want to know how you were getting on, and you didn't want to say. I remember my sister being really upset that I hadn't told her that I was going through another attempt, so she only knew when it was unsuccessful and I was really upset and all the rest of it, and I think that she felt a bit let down, or disappointed, or sad or whatever. The thing is, it was just too exhausting to confide in people, because then you had to keep them up to date or let them know.

The process of fertility treatment can put pressure on even the best relationship. Clare C talked earlier about the physical and emotional after-effects of her IVF treatment. Here she talks about the stress of the treatment on her husband, which has been echoed by a number of women we spoke to, and which ultimately led to Clare not having a second cycle of treatment as originally planned:

For him, really, he found it very, very stressful and he didn't like it because it was so unnatural. He hadn't been that keen, but he did it for me, and he didn't want to do it again. He had to go into a room and produce and there was a copy of *Caravan Monthly* on the table, that was all, you'd think they could at least have put *Penthouse* there. He wanted us to be together, as well, at the time, but we weren't allowed to be, I had to be elsewhere. It wasn't sexy, it wasn't romantic, and he found it virtually impossible to perform. He's quite shy, and he found it very embarrassing. But there wasn't a better way round it at the time. He just couldn't face going through that again.

This can be quite a common experience. Alison Bagshawe, of Guy's Hospital, says:

Often the decision to stop is not one person's. It may be because physically they can't face any more, but it may be because their partner says 'No more, you're not going through that again.'

In some cases, the stresses and strains of the fertility treatment can lead to a breakdown of the relationship. Fay found the IVF process brutal, and she talks here about the strain on her relationship with her husband, which ultimately led to their getting divorced:

I think we put ourselves under huge pressure with all of that, and I'm sure it had a lot to do with it, I don't think it was everything, but I think it probably opened up the fact that we didn't communicate well at this level, we certainly weren't in step with each other at this time. I think we were just out of step, out of tune, and didn't find a way to tune back into each other, and I think that was probably a lot to do with it.

Deciding when to stop

Deciding when to call a halt to fertility treatment can be very difficult, particularly if it hasn't been discussed and planned for beforehand. Alison Bagshawe of Guy's Hospital says that she sees many couples leaving the unit who are still in denial:

Some people leave here, still believing that a miracle can happen. The media have presented this picture that it can happen. And they latch on to it. They're still in that place of well ... either we'll go somewhere else, other treatments, get a second opinion, maybe there's a better technique elsewhere, maybe America's better, somewhere else is better, so they'll go to somewhere else.

For Sally and Jock, who talked about putting their lives on hold, it was the fact that there was no real prospect of success in the foreseeable future that led them to stop treatment. As Sally says:

I don't think it was a hard decision to stop the IVF, because it's just grim. You just can't go on and on putting your life on hold and putting yourself through that trauma – for how long do you go on banging your head against a brick wall?

And, as Jock says:

When we got to the end of it, we came to the conclusion that really there was no point in going on, because the same thing had happened every time, and there was no solution to that in the next 10 years. There were solutions to the first bit of the process, scientific and technical solutions, but there was nothing to fix this bit. No prospect. We talked, we got advice, there was no way that bit was near in the world of science, able to be fixed, so we stopped. I think we stopped in order to allow ourselves to live.

For Penny B, it was the combination of physical and emotional stress:

I was 40 and the effect of the drugs and the roller-coaster of emotions, I just couldn't put myself through the thing emotionally again. Building up that hope and always thinking positively, everyone kept saying think positively, I just couldn't do it, I knew I couldn't do it again. I knew I couldn't experience that despair again, the raised hopes then being dashed, I couldn't do it, I just knew. I didn't think, medically, I wasn't ovulating well and there weren't a very good stack of eggs, things like that, I just thought I can't do it.

There is no 'right time' to stop treatment. As Liz Scott of the Lister Hospital says:

When couples are considering the end of treatment, I encourage them to ask themselves a question. It's a very difficult question, because it's a hypothetical question. I encourage them to ask themselves what, in 3 years' time, they might be feeling in looking back on this period of time. Would they be looking back and thinking it's painful, where we are now, but at least we're able to move on because, looking back, it was the right thing to do at that time. To shut the door, as difficult as it was, allowed us to be now moving on in life. Still painful to think about, but quality of life, and closure was appropriate. Or, would they be looking back and thinking if only we'd done ... if only, if only. Sometimes one partner's not quite at the same place as the other, and are they going to be able to work towards a compromise in looking at what might effect closure for both of them.

CHAPTER 4
Relationship with self

There's a lot of evidence to suggest that, as women, our sense of self-worth or self-esteem comes from two main sources: our early childhood experience and our ongoing experience of success or failure, in whatever way we define it.

Hilary Mantel, in her autobiographical book *Giving Up the Ghost*, talks movingly about the way we define ourselves in early childhood:

> *When you were a child you had to create yourself from whatever was to hand. You had to construct yourself and make yourself into a person, fitting somehow into the niche that in your family has been always vacant, or into a vacancy left by someone dead. Sometimes you looked towards dead man's shoes, seeing how, in time, you would replace your grandmother, or her elder sister, or someone who no one really remembered but who ought to have been there: someone's miscarriage, someone's dead child. Much of what happened to you, in your early life, was constructed inside your head. You were a passive observer, you were the done-to, you were the not-explained-to; you had to listen at doors for information, or sometimes it was what you overheard; but just as often it was disinformation, or half a tale, and much of the time you probably put the wrong construction on what you picked up. How then can you create a narrative of your own life? Janet Frame*

compares the process to finding a bunch of old rags, and trying to make a dress. A party dress, I'd say: something fit to be seen in. Something to go out in and face the world.

However well we construct our party dress, or public persona, few of us enter adulthood with an internal sense of self-worth that is as good as we would like it to be. As adults many of us feel the need to go back and revisit our early childhood assumptions about ourselves to see whether we still believe them, or whether there is an alternative interpretation of our childhood experience that we can now choose to make with the benefit of our adult knowledge. And often the spur to do this is when we don't achieve something that we assumed we would, presenting a further challenge to our sense of self-worth.

Feeling a failure

As baby boomers, the 'having it all' generation, we set ourselves very high expectations of success in both our professional and our personal lives. So when we don't succeed at something as important, fundamental and normal as having a child, it can have a potentially devastating impact on our sense of self-worth.

For me (Rachel), the biggest disappointments in my life have been failing the 11 plus and not having children. It may seem ridiculous to lump the two together, but both were about failing at things I desperately wanted to accomplish and which everyone around me seemed to do effortlessly. Both deeply affected my sense of self.

It's taken me a long time to realise that everyone has their own deeply felt, personal failures. I'm coming to see that while my failures will leave scars, it's up to me whether I let them define me for the rest of my life. Very slowly, I'm learning to accept that these are things that happened to me, they're not me. After all, it's over 40 years since I flunked my exam, and 15 years since I knew I'd never have children. Changing my focus from what I haven't achieved to what I have, and more excitingly what I might achieve, is liberating, and makes me feel lighter, as if I've shed pounds.

Where our experience of not having a child is bound up with either not having a partner, or splitting up from a partner, this can reinforce our sense of personal failure. For me (Louise), in my bleaker moments, when I was without a partner, this had as much impact on my sense of self-worth as not having a child. Fay's second marriage ended in divorce after unsuccessful IVF treatment:

It was bad enough being divorced the first time, because it was a huge stigma the first time, but then to be divorced a second time, and not manage to have children. ... For a long while it felt like I was carrying a sack, I don't know whether it was a sack of sorrow or just a ton of bricks. For a while, I just felt that was how I was captioned, you know, twice divorced, no children, complete failure.

Comparisons to our friends and family can also highlight our sense of failure, particularly for those who are very competitive. Marilyn is a family doctor who is obviously well liked and well respected in her local community. She spent the first five years of her current relationship trying to get pregnant:

I think it's very difficult. I find the world is full of mothers, friends of my age who are mothers, saying how wonderful life is and how lucky they are with their children, they live for their children coming home, all the things that go around children and families. I've got a brother and a sister who've both got three children and I always feel disadvantaged. Just because they've got loving families surrounding them.

I've got a lot of friends, a lot of emotional support, but I just feel like a second rate citizen. I'm quite competitive, so I feel I've failed. I've been given these talents that I haven't used, these ovaries and all these eggs that you've never managed to use, you're so stupid. Being surrounded by my family tends to hinder rather than help. It makes me feel like a spare part, it makes me feel unsuccessful, I haven't achieved anything, I'm a failure, the black sheep kind of thing.

I just think I'm missing out; it's my competitive thing coming in. I have missed out on something major in life. All my instincts tell me to try and achieve something, rather than just accept the fact that one's failed. I'm not too keen about failure.

And the language of fertility clinics really doesn't help. Penny B tried IVF following an ectopic pregnancy, which ruptured one of her fallopian tubes (a laparoscopy having already identified that her other tube was blocked):

Even the language they used was very in your face. I remember them saying you had to reach a certain level of oestrogen before they'd harvest the eggs, and they said something like 'you've failed to reach your oestrogen level'. So it's like personal failure, and that on top of the other failure to have a baby, and failure to have an open tube, it's awful. I felt second class, and inferior and just like a failure. That's how I felt a lot. I'm a failure.

However we are feeling, we tend to pick up on the signals from the outside world that reinforce that feeling. So if we are already feeling a failure, it's the messages about failure from the outside world that we will hear and remember, making it even tougher for ourselves.

Penny B has successfully moved on. Since stopping IVF, she has had counselling, has become involved with the Chernobyl Children's Project, has strengthened her religious beliefs, and she and her husband have talked openly (at their church) about the impact of secondary infertility on their lives. She now doesn't feel the same way.

Now I don't feel a failure, I feel I've done the best I can, and that's fine. It's a bit like trying an exam, you know, you tried your best and you might get whatever exam result, but the fact that you tried your best is all that counts. It's good enough.

I have a friend who's always beating herself up about what she doesn't do, and it just drives me nuts. She's a single mum and she's got fantastic kids, but she's always looking at the 20 per cent that she hasn't achieved rather than the 80 per cent that she has achieved. I think I was there. I want to just encourage her to look at the 80 per cent, I know that's what I do now. I suppose it's fulfilment, I'm fulfilled in what I do. It might not be the picture that I had in mind, but I think there's a whole different new picture, and it's fun finding out what the new picture is going to be.

Feeling powerless

Feeling powerless or out of control about our childlessness, in contrast to the control that we exercise over other areas of our lives, is strongly linked to this sense of failure.

I (Rachel) knew that I was up against a brick wall, that there was absolutely nothing I could do to make Douglas change his mind. I felt totally powerless. Nothing in my life had prepared me for this. From an early age, I'd been encouraged to succeed, but I don't recall ever being given guidance on how to cope with failure. Finding myself in my late 30s, early 40s with no idea how to cope with my situation was frightening.

Most of us grew up believing that we could or even should be in control of our lives, and the experience of wanting a child and not being able to have one forces us to face the reality that there are parts of our lives that we can't control. Fay, who talked about being captioned as 'twice divorced, no kids, complete failure', also talks about her experience of not getting pregnant with her second husband:

Before we got married, I had this idea that I would plan it. I was teaching undergraduate students at the time, so I had decided that I would get pregnant, and the ideal time to have a baby would be at the beginning of the summer term so I could then have off the whole of the summer term, the whole of the summer vacation and be back at work for the autumn. So it was very much this was how it was going to happen. I was going to be pregnant and it would happen at this time, and of course it didn't.

So that was a very big lesson, that you can't plan certain things in life. I think I am a planner, and I am somebody who likes to think that I have a certain amount of control over what I do, and this was a huge thing. Obviously, having been through relationship break-ups, you know you don't control everything, but I think before this stage I'd felt that I could go for and do what I wanted to do. I'm a bit of a risk taker, and I take challenges ... this was a challenge I couldn't do anything about. That was initially a puzzle, and then very, very hard to realise that this was something that you had absolutely no control over.

I felt very impotent, in every sense. For me, I've been successful in other areas of my life, so to be not successful in this, everything else I can work at and do and I can make it happen, I just ... I suppose after the IVF I thought I obviously can't work at this and do it.

As well as feeling powerless about the situation, it can also feel tremendously unfair. Sally spent 5 years trying to have a baby including four unsuccessful cycles of IVF:

I've worked hard for everything, and we were brought up to believe that hard work had its rewards, and that if you were bad, God would punish you, and therefore if something really bad happens, then you're being punished, or that there's some kind of reason, and none of that applies to this, because you can try really, really hard, you can do every-thing right, but you don't get rewarded. It's like not exactly a puzzle, but the normal rules don't apply. You try and find a reason, but of course there isn't a reason. You do try to search for a meaning in it, or some kind of logic, but it's not fair, and that's how it is.

It can be really difficult for us to accept that, actually, there are areas of our lives where we aren't all powerful and in control, and where hard work alone will not make the difference between success and failure. Like Sally, we need to reach the point of being able to accept that life isn't fair.

Self-blame

When, contrary to all our expectations for our lives, we feel that we have failed in something as basic as having a child, it is very easy for this feeling of failure to turn into self-blame.

One of the most common expressions used by the women we talked to was 'feeling stupid', and it's extraordinary how many different forms this can take and the range of underlying emotions that this simple expression appears to cover.

For Judy it takes the form of feeling stupid for getting her priorities so wrong. She is a corporate vice-president in a multinational corporation, and didn't start trying to have a child until she was 42:

I think (the most important thing for me is) the sense of loss. Of not having understood how profound a human experience having children is, particularly to women, and having, through creeping non-choice, missed the opportunity. So I'm responsible for it.

I could say 'But look how blessed you are, you've got nine nieces and nephews, you've got three brothers', and then I go back to the thing I referred to earlier which is yes, you prioritise family very highly, Judy, and you love it, and you're very proud and feel privileged that you've got such a great family.

And then I say 'How do you think families are created, dummy, people have kids.' Then I'm thinking 'Oh God, how could you have got that so wrong. You won't be building any traditions, you won't be doing anything.' Even if we do it now, it'll all be wrong and disjointed, we'll be old, and I just think 'Oh crikey, how could you have not understood any of that, and why?'

Marti is menopausal following recent chemotherapy for breast cancer. Up to that point, she was still nurturing a small hope that she might get pregnant naturally, following unsuccessful fertility treatment in her late 30s. Here she talks about feeling stupid for not realising that she was leaving it too late:

I have to say the one thing I do regret hugely, and the one thing I do say to people now all the time, who say 'Yes, I want to have children,' I say 'Well get on with it before you're 35.' Because when you're 35, your fertility falls off a cliff.

And I had no idea. No bloody idea. My body was totally functional, you know periods, all that stuff, exactly as normal, and I thought all I have to do is stop using the condoms and we'll get pregnant. And we didn't. It was only when I then went to see the gynaecologist, and he then said, 'Well, you do realise ...' and I said what do you mean, I'm not having the menopause, what's this about? Anyway, duh, I didn't know.

And Marti is not alone in this. It's amazing how many women we have spoken to who are in their late 30s or early 40s, and who genuinely believe that it's simply a matter of finding the right partner, or persuading their reluctant partner to have a child. This includes women who are highly educated, intelligent and well read and whom you might assume would be better informed. There is such a low awareness of the fertility problems experienced by women over 35, coupled with an assumption that you can get pregnant right up to the time of the menopause, and if it doesn't happen naturally, well then of course IVF will solve any problems.

Sarah A's partner does not want any more children (he has two daughters from a previous marriage). She thought she had accepted the situation until an unexpected pregnancy at 42, ending in a miscarriage a short while later, brought her in touch with the depth of her feelings about wanting a child:

I know what I want, I want my partner's child or I don't want any child, and I wish I'd done this a long time ago. The net result is that I just feel stupid, I really feel stupid, I feel that's why I can't talk to anybody about it. I feel how did I, an intelligent woman, who knew this right from the word go, end up in this? I really do feel ridiculously stupid, and there are too many reminders, there are too many articles on television and radio about how to have a child when you're however old you are, as though it's every woman's right...

I feel as though I've failed as a woman. What was I here for? I wouldn't have liked in my 20s the idea that you're only here to produce children, but now I look back and it's the annoying things of how many months have you struggled through with extra doses of paracetamol because you've got really bad period cramps, and marked in your diary the days that you expect might be really bad, not to have an important meeting, and now are facing the idea of menopause, and what effect that might have on managing day-to-day meetings and ... all for nothing.

One angry thing I said to my partner at one point, 'If I'd thought when I had my first period that I would never have children, I should have just been sterilised then!' But I do feel stupid, how did I not see this coming? How did I not do something about it?

So for Sarah, and many others, the fact that you feel that it's your own fault makes childlessness particularly difficult to talk about, and for some women this is expressed as embarrassment, or shame. Like Sarah, Lara finds it very difficult to share her feelings:

I'm embarrassed, if I'm honest, I don't want to broadcast the fact that I haven't got children. I'm embarrassed, I'm ashamed, great psychotherapist that I am, because I feel that it's something that is so fundamental. So I don't find it a subject I would willingly talk about, unless somebody else wanted to talk about it. Because it's a normal thing that women do. A normal function. And we haven't quite got there, and I think that's why it's shaming.

Feelings of guilt for our earlier actions are not unusual. Kay is currently awaiting a divorce from her partner of 17 years:

Within a year and a half of knowing him, I got pregnant and it was really bad circumstances – we had nowhere to live, he was unemployed, he was only 19. So it was a bit of a sad decision, but I decided to have a termination. Which I do think about, quite a lot. I think, 'This child would be 16 now', or whatever, there's not a day that doesn't go by where I don't think about it. At the time it was something I had to do because of my circumstances.

[What stays with me] is the fact that I lost the child and it was my choice to lose it. There's a bit of guilt there, as well, I do feel a little bit guilty, but I don't regret it, if that makes any sense, I had to do it at that time, because it was the only thing I could do in my circumstances. But yes, it's not an easy thing to go through.

It can even feel as if our childlessness is a punishment for our earlier actions. Eve had two unsuccessful cycles of IVF in her late 30s:

One thing that did happen to me when I was 27, I found myself pregnant, I was having a relationship with a man who had been told that he couldn't have any children, or so he told me, anyway. I think it was a bit of a fib. I got pregnant, and I was horrified, because I wasn't very happy in this relationship and my career was just beginning to take off, so I thought this is the last thing I need. I had absolutely no qualms about having an abortion whatsoever, I did it, it was all done and dusted.

It was fine, I just got on with my life, and then when all this happened, I suddenly thought maybe I'm being punished. But then I'm not a particularly religious person, so I couldn't really think this was God punishing me, because I don't believe in God, so it couldn't be him punishing me, but I did go through a phase of thinking I'm a bad person because I had an abortion and this is my reward for it. But I don't think that any more. That was just a phase I went through.

Most people reading this book would not blame Judy or Marti or Sarah or Lara or Kay or Eve for the situations they find themselves in, yet they all blame themselves in some way. Other women we've talked to blame themselves for their childlessness, feeling that they made it happen by not wanting a child enough. Why are we all so much harder on ourselves than we are on other people? Sometimes, however difficult it may be, we just have to accept that we did the best (or the only thing) that we could do in the circumstances.

Not feeling like a real woman

For many of us, our feeling of failure is often expressed as not feeling like a 'real woman'. Despite the idea of 'having it all', there is a niggling sense for many of us that work is not as important for women as childbearing. Kathryn is single and in her early 40s:

I think that underneath it all is the belief in a lot of people, probably including myself, that really to be a woman is not to do with your job, and your status, and what you do, but with whether you have children. I've been thinking about this in terms of the pros and the cons, that it's an antiquated idea, and if you're buying into 'You're not really a woman until you've had children', then it's just taking a really simplistic view, and it's negating all the things that people have done without children, and it's also not taking into account the unhappy lives that some people have through having children, through having settled for that marriage and becoming mum, and losing your identity to some extent.

I can't instantly think of an excellent childfree/childless role model, and I think that means that somewhere deep in me I'm saying you're not a complete woman without having children, which is not what I believe logically at all, but I think emotionally I must do.

This battle between what we think, logically, and what we feel, emotionally, can be a real challenge.

For many of us, not feeling like a real woman is to do with a sense of our vital reproductive organs being unused, or redundant. Many of the women we talked to, when asked about their self-image, used words such as barren or sterile – one woman said movingly, 'I can't help feeling that women were born to reproduce. Sometimes I have a feeling of being a fruit on a tree that's withered before it actually ripened, before it reached its full potential.'

Angie is single and in her early 40s. She has never particularly wanted to be pregnant or to give birth, although she thoroughly enjoyed her experience of 'co-parenting' her ex-partner's children, and says she would now find someone with children more attractive as a potential partner than someone without. Despite her attitude towards pregnancy and giving birth, she still has a feeling of not being a proper woman:

Somewhere in my mind, still, if I never actually use this set of organs, if they work, somewhere I still feel a little bit, it's like something's not been used. Barren's not the right word ... I look at all my friends who've had babies, and parented full time, and they're fecund, that's the word for them. From what I can see, there's this extraordinary relationship with your body, and what's in it, and then what it produces, there's the baby, and then there's milk, and I suspect there's all sorts of other horrid things. Somewhere lurking in me is a sense of 'I'm not a proper woman' I guess, if I haven't had a baby.

Another aspect of not feeling like a real woman can be a very negative attitude towards your own body. Fay has already shared her feelings of being powerless when she was unable to get pregnant, and here she talks about feeling unwomanly:

I went through a real phase of feeling very unwomanly. You'd go out and about and you'd see a pregnant woman, or somebody with three children and another one on the way, and you'd think 'Hang on a minute, it's so basic, they can do it, why can't I do it? People spend all their time trying not to get pregnant, so how come now I want to get pregnant I can't?' And a huge blow to my confidence, I think, because it just felt, 'Well why can't I do this? And what do I have to do to make it happen?'

Lara, who shared her feelings of embarrassment and shame, and her unwillingness to discuss being childless, talks about her body:

[I feel] barren. I think what the bloody hell am I going through all this menopausal crap for, honestly, when I haven't even produced a baby? I do, I think all these years, and now I'm getting flushes, I'm getting the whole works. What for?

If someone looks at me and doesn't see a mother, I'm distressed. I want to be seen as if I had been a mother, or was a mother. I don't want to be seen as a single woman. Not a real woman means that you've got these breasts, and what are they doing? Sagging. Come on, they're there for feeding, and how is it that we're going to go through our life and not have that experience. I think that's what I meant when I said if someone doesn't think I look like a mother. I would like them to think that I have, and I think therefore when the person says I'm only half a woman, I would agree with that, because it's like she's a woman, she could have an affair with a guy, but what about the part of her that could be mothering? Where's that gone?

But not all women feel this way. Sally, who talked about her feelings of the unfairness of childlessness, talks here about feeling let down by her body but also about how she doesn't feel less of a woman because of it:

I haven't thought about this for a while, but I did used to feel that my body had really betrayed me, let me down, because that was another thing, if you work hard you'll be rewarded, I haven't particularly abused my body, fair share of drinking and smoking and whatever, but I've always been quite sporty and fit, and then this comes along, and it's completely unexplained. I remember looking at my body and thinking it's really let me down, and feeling quite betrayed by it, but not equating that to being more or less of a woman.

I don't feel barren or sterile; I just feel that my tubes are blocked. It's a mechanical problem, there's nothing wrong with the rest of my functioning; it's just that this passageway is gummed up. It's such a minute, stupid thing that you feel that you could somehow overcome it, you just need a bypass. It's like the motorway is blocked, so we'll just take this road and go round the other way. I don't actually see it as anything broader than that. Maybe it helps to have an explanation.

For a long time while I (Rachel) was struggling with my childlessness, I didn't feel like a real woman. I never wore skirts or dresses because they made me feel like a man in drag. I think my feminine side felt too vulnerable, too wounded to be exposed. Rationally, I knew that Douglas's rejection of children had nothing to do with me, but deep down I felt personally rejected, as if I somehow wasn't good enough. So I buried my femininity beneath a strong, sporty, asexual persona, and I'm only now just beginning to redicover it.

Other women have expressed similar feelings about their femininity. Habie is in her early 40s, and has had three failed pregnancies during her seven years of desperate attempts to have a child with her partner. She talks here about not feeling like a woman during her fertility struggles, but also about how that is now starting to change:

When I was in my teens and 20s I was a sexual woman, I had sexual partners, I could be attractive to people who liked the kind of looks that I had, and so on. Then I started to put on weight, and I was less attractive, so then it depended on the mood I was in. In the last seven years of fertility struggles, I haven't felt like a woman for a single second, until just recently, a few months ago, I've started to feel again, a little bit, like a woman, just a little bit. But I didn't, no one ever looked at me in the street, or whistled, or smiled, or said hello, or flirted at parties, ever. Because I projected an image of 'Don't touch me, I'm trying to have kids, I'm not a woman.'

But it's coming back, both the sex life and my sexuality. I went to a wedding recently, my cousin's wedding, and I made a speech, and I bought a beautiful, flowing pink dress that was very sexy and very feminine, and even though I'm overweight it somehow looked good. I made this speech and dozens of people came up afterwards to compliment the speech, and some of them were men, and they were very flirty. Twice I was chatting to a young man and people came up and said 'Oh, is this your partner, Habie?' and the man both times, a different man, said 'Oh I wish', you know, jokingly, but that has never happened to me in all these years of fertility – feeling fat, feeling ugly, feeling pregnant, feeling not pregnant.

You know when I was pregnant I didn't need men, I had my baby, my man ... and when I was not pregnant I was bereaved. Bereavement is not attractive, and nor would you want it to be, because you're self-contained in your world of bereavement. So I didn't feel like a woman at all. And now it's coming back, and I think it might just change everything. I read that women are in their prime in their 40s and I never believed it, but I'm beginning to feel like I can, the way Cuban women walk, however fat they are, they just saunter, and I went into town the other day and I sauntered, and men reacted immediately, they just do react immediately. Even before I get back a body that I feel I can be proud of, it's all in the eyes.

The sense of not feeling like a real woman has also been expressed as feeling a lack of the normal maternal instinct. As Sally, who talked about her feelings of unfairness and feeling let down by her body, says:

I don't see myself as maternal and caring in a way that a lot of mothers are, because I'm not a mother. In terms of my own self-image, it's a bit hard as opposed to soft.

Helen's husband had a vasectomy before they met. Although they have jointly decided that he will not have the vasectomy reversed, Helen still worries about not feeling like a real woman if she doesn't have children:

Sometimes I worry about, it's back to this I've made the decision not to have children, not to go through the required steps to have children, so is there something wrong with me? I do sometimes think that. If I had more of a burning urge, whatever this burning urge is, but if I had one, then maybe I would be willing to jump off the cliff, and reverse the vasectomy or whatever. (It sometimes worries me that I haven't got the burning urge) because I suppose you think you ought to have it. That somehow if you haven't got one, then you're a sandwich short of a picnic, in terms of being a real woman.

I (Rachel) feel there's a hole in my life, a chunk missing, a bit that's incomplete. It's very subtle, a physical sensation rather than a feeling. It's hard to say precisely what it's about, a lot of things I think – having a womb that's never been occupied, never being a mum, an unfulfilled dream, a decision made for me ... It's always there, like it's part of me, which feels an odd thing to say about a hole.

For me (Louise) it comes back to the challenge that Kathryn talked about earlier – logically, we don't think that we need to have children to be real women, but emotionally, there seems to be a part of us, however small, that feels that to be the case. For me the important distinction to make is between wanting and needing – however much we may have wanted to have children, it doesn't mean that we need to have children in order to be real women.

Feeling immature

Many women also express their feelings of failure in terms of feeling immature, or not feeling grown up yet because they haven't had a child. Clare A is in her late 40s, and has been married for 21 years:

I think if you never have children, in a funny sort of way you never quite grow up. I know lots of people have in their head an image of what age they are, and it's quite instructive when you ask people, 'Well in your head, what age do you think of yourself?' A lot of people will say, 'Oh, I've always been 35' or whatever. I think I've always been 17, and I think I still am. I would imagine that would have changed if I'd had the responsibility for someone else.

It manifests itself as a slight fecklessness, hopeless with money, a slight tendency to go out of my way to shock people. A sort of teenage persona that hasn't quite gone away. I think that's fair to say. Slightly sort of out to find my place in the world, which means you haven't quite got there, doesn't it?

Rebecca B, who is in her late 30s, feels as though she is stuck in a particular life stage and doesn't know how she will move forward if she doesn't have children:

I often feel as though I've got kind of stuck, you know. You go through life and life has a kind of pattern, you go to school, you go to university if you do that, you get a job, you buy a house, what's the next thing? Do I just go on as I am for the next 20, 30 years until I retire? If we really did, in the end, decide not to have children, I think that is something I really would struggle with. I feel I need to change something in my life, and if it's not that it would have to be something else and I don't quite know what.

For Kathryn, who talked earlier about her sense that for women work is not as important as childbearing, it's about missing out on adult rites of passage:

I think I don't feel grown up. My sisters (who have children) feel to me more adult, more finished than I do. I still feel that I'm stuck in some sort of limbo ... maybe it's adult rites of passage, or something like that, I haven't got married, I haven't had children ... I do sometimes think to myself that there's something wrong with me, for feeling unfinished.

When we're all together, I do sometimes feel like I'm the youngest daughter just out of school, instead of the eldest. Although we're so close in ages, it's never been a big deal. The fact that I'm the eldest makes me feel that life's passed me by, really.

Yet we shouldn't forget that there can be a real upside to not having children. Many of the women we talked to discussed feeling more youthful, and having more time, energy and fun than their peers who are mothers.

Sally, who talked about her feelings of failure and being betrayed by her body, also talks about the upside of her situation compared to her friends:

On a positive front, I'm more youthful than some of my friends, not so bowed down by some of the cares of motherhood. I think that a lot of parents fall into a kind of clichéd or well-worn relationship with their kids, where they're saying 'No you can't do that,' there's a kind of response to what's going on, whereas if you're not permanently in charge of children you can say, 'That sounds like a good idea,' you're not trying to manage them, so you can be less controlling, I see a lot of controlling behaviour by mothers.

I suppose that not having children allows you more freedom and independence, and time for yourself, and time for self-expression, all those things, and parents don't have that luxury necessarily, and it can make you more selfish, because you don't have to put other people first.

I (Rachel) revel in the fact that I can buy young, trendy clothes without fear of a critical voice saying 'Oh no, Mum!' On a good day, my stomach's flattish, I don't have varicose veins, my pelvic floor is in good order and I've no stretch marks. It may not be meaning of life stuff, but they're nice perks! Similarly, several other women talked about the positive aspects of not having children in terms of their bodies, including Janet, aged 47, 'at least I haven't lost my waistline quite yet' and Eve, aged 44, 'my body has never been used for anything other than lust!'

Regaining a sense of identity and self-worth

The impact of wanting a child and not having one on our sense of self-worth can be relatively minor or absolutely huge, but it is possible to get through this. We'll talk a lot more about coping mechanisms and alternative lifestyles towards the end of the book, but for now let's hear from two women who have worked on their sense of identity and successfully defined themselves without having had children.

Liz is a lesbian in her mid-40s, and when she came out 20 years ago, she didn't feel that becoming a mother was an option for her in the society in which she then lived. She has been with her partner for 15 years:

Early in our relationship we discussed it, but the whole social environment, it would have been extremely high risk, in terms of society's acceptance of our having children. I think we also feel that it's a gift to be able to have children, and if you're going to have children, you want to make sure that all of the circumstances around, all of the external factors, as well as your own personal commitment, are absolutely at their optimal best for the sake of that child coming into the world. We felt, I think, that we would have been disadvantaging a child at that stage.

I do think, if we've come out, we've already made so many decisions about how we redefine our lives, and how we reposition ourselves, we've already made a lot of very difficult decisions, whether they've involved children or not, so the children piece is within that. I didn't come out until I was about 25 really, although I knew I was a lesbian, probably, from the age of about 8 or 9. When you come out you've thought about whether you're going to have children or not, because you now change the whole deck of cards that you're dealing with, especially when we did it. It's part of the package, it's like you've been dealt a fistful of cards, and you look at them and say they're not for me, I'm going to chuck a number of these away, I'm going to pick up some other ones that other people don't expect you to pick up…

Helen talked about feeling 'a sandwich short of a picnic' because she didn't have enough of a burning urge to have children. Here, she describes the two halves of a picture she drew for us, first, of how she has worked on her childlessness and secondly, of what it means to her now:

Two clouds and a big question mark – they look like raindrops, but they're supposed to be effort (sweat). That is there to show that I do think it is hard work, and it's not all plain sailing. I think it's the questioning yourself, who you are, why you're here, what you're here to do, it's the questioning your decisions, have you made the right decisions or not, it's the whole very grey and very bleak time that I think you have, and that you do dip in and out of too. That's the effort part.

Then over here, on this side, we have the sun and a coffee cup, and the coffee cup to me is having time that you don't have when you have children. I do think that you can get so much more out of your relationships, all kinds of things, and I guess I symbolise that with having cups of coffee with people. Even being able to do this interview – lots of people I know who have young children would find it difficult to even fit in doing something different. So it's about having time and opportunity, and about the happiness that I do genuinely believe that you can have. Sometimes it's about making yourself sunnier than you actually feel, and sometimes I think it's just genuine output from learning to be content.

I see children as just one of those things, as I say you don't have everything that you want in life, and so lots of people, even if they have got children, haven't got other things, and I think one of the absolute keys is to be content with what you do have, and you can still be very happy.

And finally, it's also worth remembering that many mothers complain of losing their own sense of identity when they do have children.

CHAPTER 5

Relationship with a partner

By deciding to stay with Douglas, despite the high price tag, I (Rachel) saw the problem of coping with childlessness as mine not his, and working through it together did not feel an option. Even now, 15 years later, there's been very little mutual sharing of our feelings around childlessness.

Initially, his 'No children' declaration threw our relationship into a kind of limbo, with us both withdrawing into our separate worlds. I found it just too painful to be close to him. I buried myself in work during the week and spent weekends in tears, feeling totally numb and exhausted. Douglas appeared as a shadowy figure hovering on the edge of my misery. My grief was all-consuming, I didn't have the energy or the desire to find out what it was like for him, though I've no doubt he was devastated at the sudden loss of the happy, vivacious wife he'd fairly recently married. We were assumed to be blissfully happy, which made me too ashamed to discuss my feelings with anyone else. I felt totally alone.

I spent a couple of years just existing. Then I'd had enough, I was tired, even bored with feeling so alone, so at sea. I wanted desperately to break free of my grief, to start living again, and try to reconnect with the man I hoped I still loved.

The breakthrough came the evening of my first counselling session. I remember it so clearly, we were in the kitchen and Douglas casually asked me how I'd got on. Given that I'd long ago given up talking to him about childlessness, I told him I'd found the place easily and liked the counsellor. He persisted and a pattern emerged that saved our marriage. Each week, I'd talk to Mrs C, my counsellor, and then relay the conversation as we stood preparing supper. There was no discussion, no judgement, and it proved incredibly healing for us both.

This process enabled me to voice thoughts, which up to then had felt too awful to even acknowledge, let alone articulate. I told him everything, absolutely everything that had been going round and round in my head for what seemed like for ever, including all the unspeakable, unbearable thoughts that had tormented me. Like how a part of me saw him as a monstrous murderer who'd killed the children we'd never have. How I hated my married name. Rachel Black felt empty, barren, sterile. I had fully expected as Mrs Black to be up to my eyes in children, instead it felt as if Mrs Black had been strangled at birth, reduced to the name I gave the dry cleaners! I told him our marriage felt a sad joke, a sham – empty, pointless and incredibly painful.

At last, I was able to start letting go of some of the grief, resentment and disappointment that I'd been carrying around for so long. It felt like embarking on a mammoth spring clean, clearing the way for a new and different life.

It was during this period that I came up with my Survival Plan. It was a three-clause contract, later expanded to four, to which I knew I needed Douglas's agreement if our marriage was to survive. The terms were simple:

- Childlessness would never be a taboo subject between us. I could raise it whenever and wherever, be it once a month, once a day, once an hour ... whenever I felt the need.
- We would have a lifestyle we couldn't possibly have if we had children (I'll discuss this in more detail later).
- When asked 'Do you have children?', I could answer 'No, my husband didn't want any.'

Douglas readily agreed. The final building block was now in place to start working on creating a positive life together. It would not be the life I'd dreamt of living, but I was just beginning to realise that that did not mean it would necessarily be less of a life.

There's no doubt that surviving those dark days has deepened our relationship, and the pain his decision brought is now part of what binds us together.

Wanting children as part of a loving relationship, creating a family together as part of a new partnership and a new life stage is a very common dream. Not being able to fulfil this dream can feel like a double loss – not only will you not be a mother, but the whole basis of the partnership and your expectations from the relationship will have to change. This can put huge pressure on even the best relationship.

When you want a child and your partner doesn't

Having to choose between the partner you love and having children can be an agonising decision. Having chosen to be with your partner, and given up the possibility of having children, it can be very difficult, if not impossible, to discuss your emotions about that decision with your partner. I (Rachel) eventually found a way to at least share my thoughts and feelings with Douglas. Not everyone feels able to do so.

Sarah A, who is a management consultant, has always wanted children, but knew from the beginning of her relationship that her partner did not want to have any more. She thought she had accepted the situation until she discovered she was pregnant in her early 40s, although the pregnancy ended in a miscarriage a short while later:

We don't seem to have properly talked it through as a subject, so it'll always come up when I'm hurting, which makes it the worst conversation, it spirals out of control. I know that I'm having a lot of conversations in my head, and he's having a lot of conversations in his head, and there are bits that come out unsatisfactorily, so we get on with the rest of our lives.

There's that horrible expression that you learn in the very early consulting situation, the dead moose on the table. Everybody talks about absolutely everything else, and nobody mentions this festering thing in the middle of the table.

So the anger, grief, pain, shame, disbelief, sense of unfairness, injustice, resentment and whatever else you may feel, remain bottled up. It can also be very difficult to discuss those emotions with anyone else (although finding a good professional counsellor can help). It feels somehow disloyal, and having given up so much for the relationship, you don't want to do anything that might damage it.

Sarah A goes on to describe her fears of how her partner might respond, if she did raise the issue:

I don't discuss it because there's this recognition that it could be self-destructive. 'Oh if that's how you feel, then go and find somebody else, I really don't want to get in your way, and if you're not going to be the person that I fell in love with and wanted to be with, if you've changed into this sad shadow of that, I'll go and find somebody else.' So it's, Sarah, don't jeopardise it.

But, of course, emotions such as these don't just fade away. They may become underlying issues in arguments about other things. Rebecca B would love to have children, but her partner is very reluctant. Although having children has not been ruled out altogether, as she approaches 40, Rebecca feels that time may be running out:

We don't row very often, we're not the kind of couple that have big spats all the time, but when we do have rows, this is almost always what it's about at some level. I'm getting older, time's running out, are we going to do this, when are we going to do it? When I think about it, I tend to get very upset because I do feel that the clock is ticking away, and once you're over 40 it gets more and more difficult.

The challenges of infertility

Even when you are with a partner whom you love very much, and you both wanted a child, it can still put huge pressure on the relationship when infertility is the issue.

Feelings of guilt and self-blame

Where childlessness is as a result of infertility, this almost inevitably, at some level, brings up the question of whose 'fault' it is. If you are the infertile one, you may well blame yourself, and feel responsible or even guilty about the fact that you are unable to give your partner the child that you both want.

Sally had four unsuccessful cycles of IVF following a laparoscopy, which identified that her tubes were blocked. She talks about her feelings of guilt towards her partner:

I felt that I had really, really let him down. I still partly feel that. My husband sees it as something that's happened to us, not something that's happened to me, I know that's what he feels. I suppose that if it was the other way round I'd feel the same, but I feel a bit more that it's something that's happened to me, and that I've really let him down.

I did say to my husband would he be better off without me, would he like a divorce, because you feel you have to say that. I don't mean that lightly, you feel that he could start again, I haven't come up to scratch, throw me away and start again.

Having the courage to articulate her fear, and being reassured by her partner that he didn't feel that way, helped Sally slowly let go of her guilt.

Perhaps you fear that your infertility is a direct consequence of your own earlier behaviour. The sexually transmitted disease chlamydia, in particular, can be related to the age at which you became sexually active and the number of sexual partners you have had. It often goes undiagnosed in women, and is increasingly linked to female infertility. This can make it very hard not to blame yourself, and feel responsible for the infertility you are now facing.

Perhaps you had an abortion when you were much younger because the circumstances at the time were wrong, and assumed that you would be able to have a child later, in the right relationship, or the right environment. Discovering that you are now unable to have a child can bring up huge regrets and sadness, or even the feeling that you are now being 'punished' for your earlier decisions or actions. However much our rational self dismisses such ideas as fantasies, they can still prey on our minds and increase feelings of guilt and shame.

Blaming your partner

Where it is your partner who is infertile, on the other hand, it can be very hard not to blame them, or resent them, or feel that you have been given a raw deal.

Jane B had always assumed that she would have children, and after three years of trying to get pregnant unsuccessfully, she started infertility tests. When, after a further two and a half years, her husband was finally tested, it was discovered that he was infertile:

I think for a while I felt very resentful, that I was unlucky enough to have got the one that fired the blanks. It's that sort of feeling, but it isn't actual blame.

My husband and I have never, ever discussed it. I don't know whether I didn't discuss it to protect him, and how he felt, because I think I felt it was going to be easier if it was assumed that it was my problem.

I think he would say that it's ... well, I don't know what he'd say really because it's not discussed. It's not spoken about. It's sad really, isn't it, all these things? I'm sure I haven't talked to him a lot about it because I didn't want to put the blame on him. I actually don't know how he's felt about it all really, I have no idea.

Needing to protect your partner

In talking about male infertility, many of the women we spoke to reported how difficult a subject this was for their partners to discuss, striking as it does at the core of their manhood.

As Sammy Lee, a scientific consultant at the Portland Hospital, says, in his contribution to *Inconceivable Conceptions*:

> *Men avoid talking about their infertility. Where workmates or friends know about 'it', cruel jokes follow: 'I hear you are firing blanks.' Graffiti suddenly appear on toilet walls offering help with 'servicing' the wife. It is only 'boys' talk', but it may sometimes be a bitter pill to swallow. (...) Like women, men also suffer from loss of self-confidence, a feeling of incompetence, a feeling of failure, isolation, guilt, anger, shame, bitterness and frustration, when they are struggling with male infertility.*

You may well find yourself feeling the need to protect and shield your partner, at the same time as dealing with your own grief.

Following the birth of her only daughter in 1970, Linda never went back to using contraception. She assumed that she would get pregnant again, but she never did. After two or three years of inconclusive tests, she suggested that her husband be tested:

So they did, they tested his sperm and found that it was very low in motility, I think was the word they used, and they just said basically to carry on, there wasn't much else they could do. I was absolutely devastated by the whole thing, and it kind of put a finality on it, that not only was I not going to have six children, I wasn't even going to have two.

I felt as though I had to protect him, I never talked about it, I never mentioned it, I never said a word to anybody. I just said I didn't want any more children, that we had decided that one was enough with our lifestyle. I felt terrible, I felt as though I was lying all the time.

I've since spoken to other people who've been told by their doctors when they've found out that their husbands have a low sperm count, not to tell their husband. I think that's extraordinary. So they never did, and the husband went through life not knowing that it was his fault, assuming or pretending that it was the wife's fault. That wasn't my situation, but it was sort of self-imposed. I did tell him, but I then went on to protect him from anyone else knowing.

Shared experience

Sometimes, where the infertility is not immediately attributable to either partner, this can make the situation easier to bear, particularly when the diagnosis happens early on in the relationship.

Mary and her husband celebrate their golden wedding anniversary this year. After five years of marriage, they had a full range of infertility tests, which were inconclusive:

I think it brought us closer together, actually. I'm sure it did, because it was a problem we had between us. Neither one was to blame; neither of us had made a decision not to, or not to want. We just felt the same way. And we'd say oh aren't we lucky that we don't have to worry about getting babysitters, and things like that, I suppose that was a coping method as well.

Difficulties in discussing childlessness

Even within the strongest relationship, discussing infertility and the prospect of remaining childless can be very challenging. Again and again we have heard how women want to talk, but men find it very difficult or futile, and how women want to discuss how they feel, whereas their men want to talk about what to do. Eve found talking to her husband about her fertility treatment difficult:

I did feel very much on my own, really, I didn't feel I was able to talk to him about it. I told him what it was that I had to do, but he didn't seem terribly interested in it. It wasn't that he wasn't interested, he just found it quite difficult, I think, and he found it really hard to talk about.

Sarah A, whose partner doesn't want any more children, explains the problem:

If I bring it up, my partner will want to solve it, within the next half-hour, we're going to work out what the answer is to Sarah wanting children. Whereas I just want to be able to talk about it, to say it's something that hurts, but I'm working at it, and how are we going to get through it.

And Clare A says, about the diagnosis of her husband's fertility:

We certainly don't sit down and discuss it at length, and haven't, really, since it first happened. Such discussions as we had tended to be, 'Right, what can we do next, we can adopt, we can try AI', rather than 'How are we then going to live with the fact that this isn't going to happen?' We didn't really, I think, ever have that discussion.

There is an interesting insight into one man's perspective in the book *Sweet Grapes: How to Stop Being Infertile and Start Living Again*, written by Jean and Michael Carter:

> *Mike's turn: I also used to be the strong and silent type. You know, the kind who confuses silence with profundity. Actually, I was usually just unsure of myself. I didn't know how to respond to issues that presented difficult choices, so I found it easier just to withdraw. Somehow the choices would be made for me by circumstance, or more often would be taken away altogether. Either way was more comfortable than having to deal with a problem. But on the other hand, I was also a problem solver, particularly if it was someone else's problem. If, for instance, Jean would come home complaining about something that happened at the office, I would go into problem-solving mode. 'Okay' I would say 'let's look at this from another angle and see if we can find some solutions.' Or, and this is even worse, 'Sure it's a bad situation, but let's look at what you can learn from it.' I never could understand why she would get so angry. I was only trying to help. It took me a long time to learn that I really wasn't helping. Both of my strategies – silence and problem-solving – were actually ways of keeping problems at arm's length. At that distance, I didn't have to feel them. I didn't have to be a part of the hurt and confusion that come with tough issues.*

Beyond the diagnosis

Having been diagnosed as infertile, you then face a series of agonising decisions about fertility treatment, adoption or surrogacy, and we'll talk about these in detail later. Most good relationships are based on compromise, yet these are not decisions that are open to compromise – they are black and white, yes or no.

For many of the women we talked to, the biological origin of their child, or the process they would have to go through to have it, seem relatively unimportant when set against the unimaginable alternative of not having a child. For their partners, on the other hand, the processes can seem very alien, and where it won't even be your own biological child at the end of the process, this can just seem a bridge too far.

Ultimately, many women end up having to accept a decision that isn't completely their own, and that in itself can result in ongoing resentment and a sense of unfairness. As Linda, who talked about feeling the need to protect her husband from his infertility by never talking about it, goes on to say:

I think I was very resentful, not of the fact that his sperm count was low, but the fact that he didn't want to do anything about it. The fact that pride was more important than either adopting or going for infertility treatment.

The additional challenge of stepchildren

On the face of it, stepchildren may appear to be a potential 'solution' to the 'problem' of childlessness. However, in reality, the existence of stepchildren within a relationship usually creates additional pressures.

The mere fact that your partner already has what you so dearly want can be difficult to live with – it may not be jealousy, nor resentment, more a continual reminder that life isn't fair. We've heard a number of times from Anne B who gave birth to a very premature son, who only lived for 24 hours. Her husband has two children from a previous marriage:

We never really fell out about it, but the difficulty is I wouldn't accept that my husband felt as bad about it as I do. Because he says to me, 'You think it's only you, but it's not, it's my baby as well, so I feel just as bad.' Which he did. But I say 'Yes, it's different for you, because you've got children, I haven't, so to me it's double, because I've lost a baby and I still haven't got a child.' He said 'It is, it's the same.' But it's still not the same as far as I'm concerned.

The presence of stepchildren can also be a continual reminder of what is absent in your own life.

Lucy A's stepson is almost 10, and although he lives with his mother, he spends a considerable amount of time with his father and Lucy:

My own situation was compounded by the fact that I have this stepchild that the mother was trying to turn against me so much, and however much you cared for it and loved it, you're not allowed to be involved. Although you're expected to look after it, and feed it, and bath it, and make sure it's got clean uniform, and make sure that if he fell over, or woke up in the night, and in the early days it was always me that got up in the night six, seven times a night, gave him his milk before he went to bed, all the things that a mother would do. And then every time he went back you had to shut the door and say, right, no longer allowed to feel anything for the next two weeks. It didn't help at all, it made it far worse.

Most of the women we talked to who have stepchildren have, at some stage, experienced feelings of anger and frustration, have felt that their partner's love for them is in some sense diluted, or felt that they were not top of their partner's list of priorities.

Helen's husband has two daughters from his previous marriage:

In the early days of our relationship, I did find getting used to him having children very difficult. I found it very hard to get used to the idea that there were these two people in his life who were really important to him. I often felt that I should be the most important person to him, and priority number one should be me, priority number two should be his children. I was very emotional about the whole thing, I only ever saw it in an emotional way; it was what I felt they were taking away from me.

It took me quite a long time to accept that actually he is 100 per cent the dad of K, 100 per cent the dad of M, and 100 per cent my husband, and it wasn't the case that there was one pie and we all got 33 per cent each. It took me a long time to accept that, because to begin with I was so emotional about it. Then I began to realise that he would actually not be the kind of man that he is, and the kind of husband he is, if he didn't really care about his daughters.

Through a lot of discussion, at times very heated, Helen and her husband have developed ways of making it work:

I've had to grow up about it, if I'm absolutely honest, and become a lot less selfish about it, and realise that it's not just about me, and my relationship, it's about him and what his needs are too. I had to accept, also, that he would be so miserable if he was not being a good father to them, so I would be then left with a very miserable husband, who would end up resenting me. But it was an absolute battle that lasted at least a couple of years before and after our marriage. You have to fight your way out of it because the whole health of your relationship depends on it.

Not allowing childlessness to destroy your relationship

Childlessness destroys relationships. Women report two main factors that are particularly important to successful navigation through the potential minefield of a childless relationship, namely acceptance and communication.

The first factor is an acceptance, by both partners, that the relationship is more important than having a child, something that may take a long time and a lot of work to achieve. But without this acceptance, it is very difficult to move beyond the resentment, the blame, the guilt, the feeling that one or other of you would be better off with someone else.

Secondly, communication is vital. For most women, in an ideal world there would be open, frank, two-way communication, talking about feelings as well as practical issues, with both partners feeling heard and supported. In reality, this rarely happens. It may be that like me (Rachel) you accept open, frank, one-way communication. It may be that there are aspects of the situation (e.g. your partner's infertility) that you will have to accept as being off limits. But even so, it's important that you are able to talk about the impact of this on you.

Lucy A was 36 when she married her second husband, and was about to start IVF when tests identified that she had cancer and would have to have a hysterectomy.

Ten years later, she still goes through bad patches:

The difficulty was, when I was in pain, my husband would see it as me being an irrational woman, as opposed to just saying 'Come here darling; let me put my arms around you.' He didn't do that; I was left on my own to go through the agony, and it was agony, it was huge pain. So I always felt very isolated. You know, he could be the most wonderful man in the world, but when it came to me needing him, at that level, he wasn't there. He just could not deal with it, he couldn't cope, he didn't understand and that did affect my feelings for him at the time.

I (Rachel) can readily identify with Lucy A's longing for support that's not forthcoming. And I've come to realise that my husband's irritation or silence at my grief stemmed in part from feelings of inadequacy, of not being able to make things better for me. So now when I need his support I make it clear that being listened to and hugged is all I need. Just being there for me physically and emotionally is enormously valuable. There is no magic wand. In fact, he's not required to say a word.

The impact of childlessness on sex life

From the moment Douglas made his 'No children' declaration, sex became an emotional minefield, and my (Rachel's) recovery has been painfully slow. Initially, I found myself vacillating between two extremes. I went through phases of totally rejecting sex, as too distressing, depressing, even pointless given its natural outcome was now denied me. Rejection was also a form of punishment. I felt angry; he needed to suffer like I was. At other times, my desire for sex appeared insatiable, though in reality my goal was to be one of the 2 per cent failure rate associated with the coil. But such tactics didn't really help me.

Sex became very confusing. To withhold sex gave me some pleasure, but at a price. It distanced me from Douglas whose love and physical closeness I desperately needed if I was to come to accept our childlessness. Yet how could I love and open myself up (literally!) to someone who had unilaterally stopped me from being a mother, something I desperately wanted? When on occasions, I enjoyed sex, I felt guilty, since such pleasure seemed a betrayal of my grief.

Of course, all this was totally hidden from the outside world. When people asked the dreaded question 'When are you two planning to start a family?', I found Douglas's jokey 'No plans, we're just practising' response sickening and very hurtful. While understandable, in that he did not want aspersions thrown at his masculinity, it totally denied my grief and our extremely fractured sex life. Part of me longed to tell the ugly truth, but my overriding pain and shame silenced me.

It was against this background and problems with the coil that I came up with the final clause in my Survival Plan (see page 100) – for Douglas to have a vasectomy.

Given the circumstances, I felt he should take responsibility for contraception, and I knew he loathed condoms. But if I'm really honest the reasons behind my suggestion were far more emotional than rational. I knew he hated anything to do with hospitals and abhorred intimate medical examinations. To agree to a vasectomy would cost him dear, and the thought of him suffering with some-thing linked to reproduction felt incredibly comforting. From a personal perspective, it would also remove the smidgeon of hope I felt every time we made love; hope which always ended in despair on the arrival of my period. I knew the pregnancy fantasy needed to be killed off if I was to move on from the pain of childlessness.

I also knew the snip for him would ensure that, if our relationship did collapse, no other woman could get what I'd given up, or at least not easily! I'm not proud of these thoughts, but I was desperate. I was fighting for the survival of our marriage. A vasectomy would mean the cost would not be all one-sided, as it had felt to date. He would be paying a price for his rejection of children and I would regain some control.

After a few weeks mulling it over, Douglas agreed and had it done. Sadly, it was many more years before I felt ready and able to rekindle my libido, but the vasectomy was an important step on the road to rebuilding our relationship.

Only recently have I finally come to accept that my husband's rejection of children arises from issues in his past, and has nothing to do with me. This realisation, together with attending a weekend Essence Foundation workshop (see Appendix 1), has finally enabled me to begin to reclaim my femininity. After years of feeling barren, sterile and rejected, I'm just beginning to rediscover my sexual appetite and it feels good.

Many of the women we talked to have spent years, if not actively trying to get pregnant, certainly hoping that they would do so. Years of taking your temperature and filling out ovulation charts, trying to maximise your chances of conceiving, can kill sexual spontaneity in the best of relationships. And, in addition, there's the long-term effect of the emotional monthly roller-coaster of waiting, hoping that you've succeeded, followed by desperate disappointment. It's a cruel irony that, over time, the desperate desire for a child can severely reduce the desire for sex, which becomes simply a means to an end, and ultimately pointless.

Natasha and her husband have one son, aged 6, and for the past four years have been trying for a second child, including various fertility treatments. She talks about the impact that all this had on their sex life:

I think it just ruins your whole libido. Your whole partnership becomes devoid of sensuality, it becomes just something about doing an act that is about a sperm meeting an egg, and that is it. The pressure was on, and the pressure was on him, and the pressure was on me and basically sex becomes like this flag going down in a race and 'You're off!' Only you lose the race, every single month.

It just takes away any of the spontaneity, any of the pleasure, I hope not for ever, but I think to a certain extent it ruined a part of that for us. I really do believe that. It closed me off to sex being anything other than something you make a child out of.

And of course the procedures associated with fertility treatments can be highly stressful. Close scrutiny of your sex life by the medical profession, daily injections, strong drugs with all their physical and emotional side effects, your partner having to provide sperm samples on demand (and not in the most conducive environments), repeated insemination with a plastic penis – even in the most sympathetic and well-run clinics, this can all be an incredible invasion of one's privacy, deeply unpleasant and distressing, or even shameful for some.

Whatever the processes you have been through, if you are unable to talk about how you're feeling, your anger, grief, resentment, blame, guilt or whatever is uppermost for you, then all this emotional baggage can have a disastrous effect on your libido.

Jane B talked about her husband's infertility, and their inability to discuss it as a couple. Here, she talks about the impact on their sex life of the years of trying to get pregnant, before the diagnosis:

The one thing that I would say is a lasting effect of trying to get pregnant is the result it has on your sex life. Certainly in our case, it's never regained the spontaneity.

I must have gone very peculiar for a couple of years; we had hardly any sex at all. My body ... I just withdrew my body. I've often wondered whether it was punishment, the withdrawal, because there was no point, he was firing blanks, what's the point? And by that time you've actually lost an awful lot of interest, because you've done it so many times with so little ... and you just do it, and you wait, and you hope. In actual fact, you're just doing it; any sort of spontaneity goes out of the window.

I don't know how, I'd love to know how people make it come back and make it right. Because I don't think they do make it right. Or at least I haven't been able to completely make it right.

Clare A talked about her difficulty in discussing the emotional aspects of their situation with her husband. Here she goes on to admit how the diagnosis of infertility has affected her view of her husband:

I think it's some kind of biological imperative that someone who you know can get you pregnant, I think you do view them differently from someone who can't. I think that does have an effect. I've seen various documentaries to do with the fact that women's natural instinct is to find the strongest gene, the alpha male, the strongest sperm, whatever. I think that is at play, you might not recognise it at first, but I think it does have an effect.

I think we have a more low-key relationship than we did. It's hard to tell how much of that is age and general overwork, but yes I think it does diminish the sexual side of your relationship, or it did in our case.

And as we have already discussed, being childless can have a significant impact on our image of ourselves as women, leaving us feeling unfeminine, failures, not 'real' or 'complete' women, and this in turn can affect our sexuality.

How to improve your sex life
One of the most important things to realise is – you are not alone.

In their book, *Reclaiming Desire*, Doctors Goldstein and Brandon estimate that low libido affects an estimated 22 to 43 per cent of the female population in the US. Based on our discussions, we have no doubt that the percentage is much higher among the involuntarily childless.

As Pauline Brown, a psychosexual therapist with Couple Counselling, Scotland, says:

We forget that the biggest sexual organ is the brain, and if the brain is focused on procreation, fertilising that egg, sexuality as such does go out of the window. Procreation becomes the key purpose for making love, rather than for the emotional as well as physical connection that sex is usually about.

The other key factor about sexuality is that we have to want to be sexual. We can, and people do, switch ourselves off, switch our sexuality off, and difficulties with fertility is often one of the areas where sexuality does seem to get switched off – 'Well, we can't make babies, so why bother?' Not all, but most, women expect to have children and if it doesn't happen, getting over that is crucial and can take years. All that loss needs to be mourned before you can even think about sex as a loving part of a warm relationship. It's too much of a burden, when someone's going through a mourning period, to expect their libido to be functioning normally.

So what can we do about it? Being able to talk about the stress of childlessness, whether to your partner, to close friends or to a counsellor, will undoubtedly help. Research shows clearly that having good support is one of the best ways of reducing the impact of stress in your life, as are good physical health, adequate sleep, regular exercise and limited consumption of alcohol. Having a routine that includes regular time for relaxing can also be beneficial.

If you suspect that your low libido is related to emotional issues that remain unresolved with your partner, it is worth considering Goldstein and Brandon's observations. Many of their clients have realised that they subconsciously use their lack of sex drive to convey their anger towards their partner, and that this allows them to release their negative emotions without direct confrontation. Yet anger is an essential part of all intimate relationships. If it isn't expressed or discussed, it can emerge in other parts of our relationships – including our sex lives. Rejecting your partner's advances is one way of taking control of the situation and letting him know just how you are feeling. On the other hand, if you were to improve your libido, you'd need to find other ways to acknowledge and address these feelings, which may be challenging.

Even if you've successfully worked through all the emotional issues, with yourself, with your partner, and have reached a point of accepting your childlessness and everything that led you to this situation, it's also important to realise that, in order to regain your libido, you will need to take some positive action – without this, your libido won't just magically improve.

As Pauline Brown says:

Sexuality is energy. Sex appeal means that somebody's sexual energy is high and is visible, perhaps more so than somebody else's. It's about nurturing that energy, and like any other energy, the physical energy that gets us going to the gym rather than slobbing in front of the TV, it really needs to be nurtured.

Pauline encourages us to spend time with ourselves sexually, and to think about sensuality, not just sexuality:

Working on the premise that our most important sexual relationship is with ourselves, when we have supported and encouraged and developed our own sexuality, and we own it and are in control of it, it's much easier to share it. It's also easier when you know what pleases and supports your own sexuality to be able to share that with a partner. All of that helps to get people back into themselves.

Don't stand in the shower thinking about the meeting that you're going to be in at 9:30 that morning, and whether you've got your notes. Stand in the shower and be in the shower. Think about the feel of the water on your body, the temperature of the water, the feel of the steam in the bathroom, the music that might be playing on the radio at that moment, what the towel that you're drying yourself with feels like, so you're concentrating on the moment. This is one of the ways that we can remove ourselves from our sensuality – some people can make love and they're thinking of the shopping list.

I encourage people to have lots of different things – I've got the nylon things, bristle brushes, loofahs, different textures, and to think about what they're doing, think about the texture, the feel on the arm, the feel on the shoulders, the feel on the breasts, the feel on the genitalia. I encourage people to get back into their sexuality being their own. We own our sexuality, we don't need someone to come along and turn it on, like a switch, human beings are not like that, our sexuality belongs to us. It's putting people back in touch, and in charge of that.

Pauline also talks about the importance of reawakening the emotional connection with your partner:

So that sex doesn't just become this thing that happens, maybe on a Saturday night for 10 minutes, but it becomes a regular part of the relationship – you might have a kiss and a cuddle while one of you is washing the dishes or stacking the dishwasher. You might sit at the dinner table and stroke your partner's hand – that's about sensuality, it's not about sex. It's almost like reawakening an emotional connection that takes into account all of our being, not just our sexuality or our fertility.

Finally, she talks about the importance of putting the romance back into sex, and considering all five senses, not just the sense of touch:

You need to put the romance back around sex. What I call the extended foreplay, which I think is getting dressed up to go out for dinner, and all the things that we do when we're courting, in the early days, you know, you're meeting your beloved that night and you make an effort, and you dress nicely and you smell wonderful, and you've made an effort with your hair, both men and women, to look attractive to the beloved, and the care and attention that we pay to the other partner for their cares and their concerns, the enjoyable dinner, the good food, the good wine, the conversation, all of that is part of the foreplay, part of the softening up. And I think we really need to go back to that. It puts the excitement and the expectation back. It's reminding ourselves of why we first fell in love with that person. It's that bit about making each other feel wanted again.

If the biggest sexual organ is the brain, it's about how we allow ourselves to switch that back on, what do we do to encourage and support that. We try and work with the five senses, so that sexuality is grounded in the whole of us, so that it's about sight and sound and taste and smell (as well as touch). We need to think about how we encourage and stroke that positively. So you have the nice dinner and then you go home, and it might be the candlelight, or soft lamp lighting or whatever you've got, the nice music that you put on the CD player to support the romantic mood. I encourage people to use scent as much as possible, so that might be scented candles, it might be incense sticks. We're encouraging all the senses, so that sex is not just reduced to the physical touch. It's getting back to sensuality, not just sexuality.

Of course, you're not going to find all the answers here, and we can't pretend that recapturing the joy and spontaneity of your pre-child-lessness sex life is an easy task, but if you really want to improve your libido, it can be done, although it may well take time and effort.

Successful relationships

However difficult it may seem, it is possible to successfully navigate the challenges of a childless relationship and couples who do succeed can often end up with very strong relationships as a result.

Eve married in her late 30s, and had two unsuccessful cycles of IVF. At the time, she found it difficult to discuss the situation with her husband, but, over time, it has become easier:

I think that our relationship's just gone that one step further now. I feel a lot more able now to say things to him, like 'I should have had a child' or 'I could have done this, we could have done that', and he'll say 'I know'. It's good that I feel that I can say these things, whereas a few years ago I'd just have thought them. I used to think it was definitely, 'Keep out, danger!', but I think I'm getting to feel it's a difficult area, but it's not a taboo any more, it's not a 'Do not enter'. I'm sure the day will come when I look on it and think 'Oh well, I've done a load of other things'. That's my hope.

Childlessness has probably made our relationship. Obviously we have a lot more time for each other, and that's what makes it so good, I think. It has definitely got better, and I think probably because we both put more into it. He's a very loving person, and he always goes out of his way to make me feel wanted, he's very demonstrative about his feelings, physically and verbally, which is great, far more than he used to be. I suppose he's aware that I've had a hard time, and I guess that's his way of dealing with it.

Lucy B was in her early 30s, and had only been married for six weeks when both ovaries were removed, and she went into an early menopause. Now, five years later, she says:

It's made us very close. We're definitely a very strong little unit, as it's just us, and that's how it's always going to be. So yes, I think it's made us very, very close. Because we do have all that time for one another, as well. We're not both tired from disturbed sleep. There isn't anybody else competing for the other person's attention. So we are very, very close. That is a very positive thing to take out of it.

CHAPTER 6

Relationships with the rest of the world

Other people's expectations

It can be hard enough to deal with our own thwarted expectations for motherhood, but we also have to deal with a whole host of external expectations. From an early age, it can feel as though we face a barrage of questions: Do you have a boyfriend? When are you getting engaged? Have you set a date yet? When are you starting a family?

Mothers often have strong expectations of their children, particularly their daughters, to have children of their own. Kay is in her late 30s, and her mother is in her late 60s:

Oh, my mother would love me to. 'Oh you're leaving it too late, you'll never have them.' She goes on a bit. I don't pay much attention to it, really, I just think it's up to me. I'm not going to have a baby just for the sake of it. It's a mother–daughter thing, isn't it. My mum's quite a mumsy mum, and I'm her youngest, and she would love me to have children. I think more for her sake. I think it's quite selfish, it's so she's got a part of me again, and it's a little something she can be mumsy with. She can't be mumsy with me any more although she still tries.

For some of us, the expectations from our mothers can be more complicated. Yes, they want us to have children (and provide them with grandchildren), but they also want us to make the most of our opportunities, opportunities that they themselves probably didn't have. Sarah A is a management consultant:

I don't know whether I thought I'd got all the time in the world, but I do think I felt that there was an expectation. My mother hadn't gone to university, my mum had been the brightest girl in the school but had left at 16 after her school certificate, because gran was widowed and needed mum to go out and work. And all the wonderful women who set up my college, these women really fought a lot to give me a lot, I really feel like I need to do something with it, I need to prove that it's worth educating a woman, we're not just going to go and cook cookies for the rest of our lives, we're going to use the studies that we've got.

When I (Rachel) told my parents about Douglas's rejection of children, they were very supportive. They were very sad for me, and respectful and admiring of my decision to stay with him. My mother is the only person ever to express sympathy for Douglas in his need to come to his decision.

My mother-in-law was absolutely dumbstruck when I told her. Being very straight talking, her immediate response was to ask 'Is his tackle all in order?' When assured that it was, she was, and still is, totally mystified and upset by his decision. She felt very strongly that it wasn't fair on me for Douglas to deny me children, it was my right as a healthy, loving wife. At one point, she suggested I might consider adopting a more relaxed attitude to contraception. Though trying to help me, her suggestion made me feel that our childlessness lay in my hands, within my control, which was hard to hear. While a 'mistake' would have given me what I really wanted, it would have been a total violation of trust I couldn't have lived with. For a long time, I felt confused and a bit resentful, as if I was partly responsible for depriving them of grandchildren, not that they ever said or probably ever felt this.

Overt pressure from fathers is less common, but that doesn't mean that there isn't still an element of expectation, as Rebecca B experienced:

There was a very embarrassing occasion a few years ago when my brother and his wife, and I think it was just me, took my father out for lunch. He had a little bit too much to drink and started getting very maudlin about the fact that he didn't have any grandchildren; this was before my sister had her children. I had the feeling that this was some-thing quite deep-seated, that he'd been trying not to pressurise us, but he really wanted them. He's absolutely mad about the two that he does have now.

Rebecca A is in her early 40s and single, and she feels the weight of expectation from her family:

In my family, I am certainly defined by my childlessness. At my aunt and uncle's silver wedding I was introduced by my grandmother to a friend of hers as 'This is the granddaughter that can't get a man'. I'm able to recognise now that I have a right to be angry about things like that, because how many other of her grandchildren have been to university, have a job like mine, are nice people, but all that mattered to her was that I wasn't married, didn't have a man, and didn't have children.

And it needn't just be our immediate family. Elaine is single and in her mid-40s:

Last year, at my youngest sister's wedding, a cousin took me aside and said 'What's the matter with you, you're 43, you're not getting any younger you know, you'd better have kids before you dry up. You're going to dry up soon, you know, so what are you messing around for?' I just couldn't believe that somebody who I've got this loose relationship with, family connection, could even dream that he had the right to speak to me like that. I can't tell you how upset-ting that was. I was enraged that he would think that he had the right to tell me what I can or can't do with my life, but I was also really upset, that that's probably how people see me, and there's probably lots of other relatives that see me as dried up, that's the words he used.

In addition to expectations from our family, we may move in social circles where it feels like everyone we know has children, and expects us to do the same. When Clare A was in her 30s, she and her husband spent a number of years trying to have children unsuccessfully.

It was very unfortunate, at that time we were living in a suburb which is now referred to as Nappy Valley. It's one of those sort of middle class young married settlement areas which was literally swarming with children. So the only topic of conversation when you were going to have a drink with a neighbour, or a party or whatever, was the latest arrival or who was pregnant. It frankly was the worse possible place to be, although obviously we'd moved there thinking that we'd be joining in.

And, of course, we have all faced that awful question when we meet people for the first time: 'Do you have children?' For the person asking, it's almost certainly just a simple, social opening gambit, like 'How are you?' or 'What do you do?', but for us it can reinforce our sense of failure, and of not fitting in.

Interestingly, other people's expectations are not just an issue for childless women – a number of the women we talked to, like Wendy, who had one child but would dearly have loved to have more, have talked about the pressures at the school gate:

You're kind of programmed into it – 'Are you going to have children?' – when you're first married. Once you've had one, you think 'Oh, thank God', but then there's this same sort of deal. 'Oh you're not just having one are you? Oh, poor only child, you can't do that.' Family, friends, people totally unintentionally, it's almost like a social norm, isn't it, 'Oh when are you having the second?', it's like 'How are you?'

In my case, you're thinking 'Are they imagining there's something wrong with me?', there's that kind of thing. Or that people would see faults in your partner, 'Oh can't you manage it?' There's all that kind of bravado, which everybody laughs at ... it's just to protect people, really. I do remember at the time, it's kind of at the school gate where all this nastiness goes on when everyone's collecting all their children.

At times, it can feel as though the whole of society is geared towards families. Since Fay's divorce ten years ago, she's been in and out of relationships, but is not in a relationship at the moment:

I still do have some resentment around the way society views you as a person without children. Part of my buying my house, which is very definitely not a family home, is about saying I'm fed up with trying to fit into what society builds for you, which is that you're either a young singleton or you're a family, in a sense. Supermarkets, everything is geared towards the big – there are huge aisles of supermarkets I don't even need to go near, because they're so vast, and everything is geared up to buying in bigger bulk, bigger packs. It's almost like you're a loser because you're just buying for you.

Media pressures

This feeling of not fitting in can be reinforced by the media. As Kathryn, who is single, says:

If you open a magazine or you read a celebrity interview, it seems to be the fashion now to get married early and have kids. I think that in the media you've still got this picture of the Victoria Beckhams on the one hand, and the Bridget Jones on the other. One is put on a pedestal and the other is seen as a bit sad, really, so I don't think that helps.

And as Habie says:

In television terms, I think the imperative for a happy ending means that all the childlessness issues in the main soaps that I've been watching for five years have ended in success. I just feel that total childlessness is never dealt with. Everyone's always got a stepchild or another child that's grown up and they want more, it's not fair, you know.

Some of us are lucky enough to have good childless role models in our lives – the eccentric aunt, our Brown Owl or Guide Captain, or our mother's glamorous bridesmaid who remained single and spent her time trotting off around the world. However, if we don't have such role models from our family and friends in childhood, then the absence of any positive childless role models in the public domain really doesn't help and can reinforce our sense of isolation and failure.

I (Rachel) have spent literally years on the lookout for prominent women who have survived wanting and not having children, and have gone on to lead happy, fulfilled lives. I needed proof that it could be done and ideally tips on how to do it, but I never found any. It's as if childlessness is something shameful to be kept in the closet. Eventually, I found a role model of sorts in my next-door neighbour, a wonderfully warm, motherly type in her mid-60s whose children had grown up and moved abroad. Her life was full, vibrant and now childfree. She provided the inspiration I sought, although our friendship felt bittersweet. Finding real kinship with a woman almost 30 years my senior reinforced how alienated I felt from my own generation, who were submerged in motherhood.

Religious and cultural expectations

We may also face additional expectations or pressures from our religious or cultural background and upbringing. Natasha, who is Jewish, has one son and would dearly have loved another child:

For me, being Jewish isn't really about the religion, so much, it's about the lifestyle and all the traditions and the community as well. It's about being brought up in a certain way. But things like the proximity of the parents means that they're in your lives more, and so because of that there's more pressure. It's not like my son only sees them six times a year, or just spends summer holidays and Easter and Christmas with them, it's more than that, they're ongoing relationships, there's lots of popping in by family. So that, I think, makes it more difficult, because we're not a family that's split over the country, or the world, or whatever.

Linda is also Jewish. She too has one child and tried unsuccessfully for many years to have more:

As Jewish kids, you're brought up to succeed, to succeed in everything and anything you do, you must succeed and it doesn't even matter what it is, but you have to be the best at it. That's part of ... you just always know that you're expected to succeed.

And so if what you want is six children then you're expected to have those six children. You get married and you are expected to marry someone successful ... failure isn't part of the game. When I said to my mother that I only wanted one, she was quite happy if that was what I wanted. But if it wasn't what I wanted, then it wasn't right.

Sue was brought up as a Catholic, and talks here about the additional pressure that she feels:

Children are very much a blessing from God and to me it was always tied into the 'You're guilty the moment you're born'. All humans are guilty, and Catholic guilt is something that you run from for the rest of your life. So if you're not blessed with children, then that's God punishing you for being guilty, or being bad. So you're constantly having this reiteration of your guilt.

Kate is a lesbian who has been trying to get pregnant by self-administered donor insemination and has now decided to adopt. She talks here of her doubts, as a Catholic:

Because I come from a Catholic background, in the newspaper the Pope had done his annual address to the people and there was a huge thing on one page, where the Pope had said 'Lesbian and gay adoption is a violence against children'. They were the words that he'd used in his address, 'a violence against children'. It was almost like ... that's it, that's what's bothering me, because I know some people think those sorts of things.

Elaine talked earlier in this chapter about a cousin calling her 'dried up'. Here, she goes on to talk about the additional pressures that she faces, being from a Jamaican, West Indian background:

I think it does add pressure, because the only people I know that don't have children from the black community are people who can't have children. Now, to all intents and purposes, if I go by that one experience that I had when I was 28 [an unplanned pregnancy], I can have children. So I think I can, as far as I'm aware, have children, but the circumstances haven't happened. So from that point of view, yes, I'm very strange.

My father was the biggest chauvinist imaginable. There was always a sense of proving him wrong, that women have more to offer than being somebody's wife and somebody's mother, because as far as my dad was concerned, that was women's sole value. They had nothing else to offer, and that's their key importance. I think a lot of his chauvinism was cultural, not just him personally, so I think the pressure comes from that. That's how many people in our community will view women – women's only value is to be a wife and a mother. There's nothing else. I think a lot of black people are still like that. So to my father, I was a complete and total failure in life. He died when I was 38 and I was single and childless.

For a woman from the Hindu or Muslim faith, having children is not merely an expectation, it's an obligation. It's her part in the marriage contract, to provide not just a child, but a male heir, to pass on the name, the property and to look after her and her husband in old age. It is widely assumed that any problems with fertility are the woman's fault. (In reality, where couples seek treatment, statistics show that approximately one-third of all infertility is attributable to the woman, one-third is attributable to the man and the remaining one-third is unexplained.)

Hira is in her mid-40s, and has been married for 12 years:

When I got married I had hopes and dreams that I would have children and I would lead a normal life. My husband has a problem, not me. If I'd got a problem, I'd be out from his life. Asian people, especially gents, they don't understand, they don't accept that there should be fault in them, all the time they think the fault is with the woman. When I came to this country, I talked to the doctor, and he said 'Did your husband check?', I said 'No'. He sent my husband for the check-up, and he said 'He has the problem, not you.' My husband never accepted it, he said 'No, I'm OK.'

Sam is in her early 40s, and has been married for eight years. She has severe endometriosis and damaged fallopian tubes:

I got more feelings when we went to Pakistan. My husband's family, they kept asking, the aunties and uncles and the cousins, all of them, about the children. They said 'What is the problem?', and 'Why doesn't it happen?', and I told them. My one sister-in-law she says, 'Why you don't say to your husband get married again?' I said to her, 'I told your brother if he wants, he can get married, because the problem is in me.'

It's usual in our culture, in our religion as well. If the lady can't give you a baby for ten years, you are allowed to get married again. Culture wise, she just said, without thinking about my feelings, she just said it clearly, 'Why you don't say to our brother to get married?' I said 'I don't stop your brother, if he wants, he can, I told him so many times, if you want babies I don't stop you, because this is the happiness you can get from others but not from me.' But my husband he's always close to me, and he says, 'If I need a happiness, I need from you, if it's not then I don't, and I'm happy as I am now.'

I got worried when I went to Pakistan, because I thought there are some of his relatives, and I had a feeling that they insisted he should get married again, and maybe his mind can change, it could happen, and this actually worries me sometimes.

Although coming from a religious background can mean that women face additional expectations and pressures about having children, having religious faith can also help women in living with their childlessness.

Paula is in her mid-50s and single, and has struggled with feeling a failure and feeling unacceptable to the rest of the world because she doesn't have children. Her religion has helped her considerably with her struggle with self-blame:

Religion is relevant to everything in my life, and I think it's helped me a great deal to get over the fact that I'm perhaps not as good as other people, or I thought I wasn't as good as other people, because I didn't have children. I used to think that, I used to think I'm just not good enough to be loved, to be married, to have children. God's love is so enveloping that he doesn't think like that. It's so out of his character, that that is very helpful.

Penny B has one teenage daughter and desperately wanted more children. She had always been a church-goer, but here she talks about how her faith helped her through a very difficult time:

I remember, it was in the autumn, it must have been 2000, a friend of mine had had a single child, a daughter, and the daughter was a couple of years younger than mine. We'd always propped each other up in the pub and confided about having onlys. She'd had a stillborn child, and she couldn't have any more. We used to compare notes, and she would say, 'It's really hard having an only, isn't it, because people make assumptions, don't they?' They actually can be quite cruel in the things that they say. We were a sort of club of mums with onlys.

Then, I was in the car park, just walking to my car, and I saw her and waved to her. I went over to her, and I can remember it to this day, she was six months pregnant. It absolutely floored me. Completely floored me. It just sort of hit me in the stomach. The thing that really upset me was that I couldn't be happy for her. I was, after the initial shock, but initially, it was just absolute, pure jealousy. Why her? Why her, why not me? All the time I was weeping inside.

A short time later, Penny saw someone in a TV documentary talking about finding complete peace through God:

And I thought 'Oh, that's what I want, I just so want that peace, I just long for it.' I remember waking up in the morning, the next morning, and thinking I've got to go and find and have this peace. What's this peace, how do you get this peace?

I found that peace, through the church, through Jesus, through becoming Christian. I'd been a church attendee, going through the motions, but actually sort of opening your heart up and saying 'Here I am ...' Sometimes you hear about people who hit rock bottom, and you actually say 'Right, I can't do this on my own.'

There's a bit in the Bible that says come unto me all ye that are heavy laden and I will give you rest. You actually dump your burden at the cross. And that's what it felt like, woomph. That jealousy, that resentment, that grief, that bitterness ... it still doesn't mean that you don't sometimes feel bits of those feelings, maybe about other things, but I don't now about other children.

And Sam, who talked about the pressure from her husband's family when they returned to Pakistan, goes on to talk about her feelings of fatalism about being childless:

Being a Muslim, we are just thankful for what God has given to us. If God didn't give me this one, maybe I'm not able to do that, maybe I'm not able to be a good mum, maybe my husband is not able to be a good father, maybe something is behind that, and that's why God didn't give me that child. If the child comes in the world, maybe something happen to the child, and God save us from this sadness and just give us a little sadness that we don't have a baby. Maybe when we get the baby, it's disabled, you will get more worries, maybe only because God knows what is good for you and what is bad for you. Always I end up with this belief. It's all in God's hands. If God wants to do it, it will happen. This makes me relax.

Other people's assumptions

Even if we can learn to live with our childlessness, as childless women we face a constant barrage of assumptions that are made about us by other people. These can be very frustrating and difficult to accept, particularly as they are often covert, not openly discussed. Nowhere is this more the case than in the working environment. Liz shares her frustration at assumptions that are made in the workplace:

I think employers, it's not particularly the case with my company by the way, although I've seen bits of it, I mean if there's something that needs to be done that's got to be done late at night, someone has to work longer hours, it's easy for them to say 'Well, you're not going home to feed the kids', or 'You don't have to take little Rosie off to Brownies', so I think it can easily be a case of 'The job's got to be done, you don't have a family, you can do it can't you?', I think there's a bit of that there. Because everybody knows that family comes first, and you don't have one, do you, so you can do the work.

Kay works in a care home for disabled adults:

We've got a couple of women who've got childcare problems at work, and a lot of them are copping the early shifts. It's OK, I understand when you have children you have commitments and you've got to work around them, but I'm childless, so I'm getting a lot of late shifts, whereas if I had a child I'd probably have a better rota. That annoys me, because I don't think it's very fair, really, I think they should make a compromise. I still have a life, whether I've got children or not, I still have a life. [The late shift is] 2:30 to 10:00, so you can't really do much with the morning. I seem to be getting it a lot, whereas the women with children are getting the nicer little slots, 7:30 to 3:00.

Sarah A, a management consultant who spoke earlier about the weight of other people's expectations, talks about the irony of being a childless professional woman in the new millennium:

Through my 20s I battled against this attitude of 'You're a woman; you're going to leave and have children'. Now in a way I'm battling against the results of that, which are people being extra concerned about women colleagues. I really wish I didn't have to put up with this,

I've covered for women with children, women on maternity leave, and whoever covers for me to do anything, what's the payback?

The classic was, I'm looking to move into a different role at the moment, so I picked up an internal project. The man interviewing me said 'Do you have any problem travelling?' and I said 'No, I've always done it.' He said 'Oh, that's good, because we've got a particularly fertile team, and 20 of our team have had babies in the last year, and I don't want them to be away from their wives.' And I thought that's really ironic, suddenly I'm the one that gets the overseas projects, because these guys want to be at home with their wives and children. So I do find a lot of very difficult things about it.

And it's not just at work – our time may be seen as less valuable in other ways. Rebecca A talked earlier about feeling defined by her childlessness (all of her siblings have children):

It's this ... the single, childless woman ends up looking after the parent, the aged parents, that I'm very conscious of now as my mother gets older. Thank goodness she's very sprightly and doesn't need me yet, but it will be assumed that it's my role. When my father died, it was me who was expected to look after my mum, it was never that my feelings were legitimate, it was always 'How is your mother?', and aunts would say 'You must bring your mother over to see us, and you can stay too' – why would I want to, for heaven's sake? But it's my duty, of course, to look after her, because I don't have anyone else to look after.

Because we don't often talk about childlessness, it can feel overwhelmingly as though we face being either pitied or judged for being childless.

Kathryn, who talked about the way the media can reinforce our feeling of not fitting in, sums this up:

I think a lot of people think 'Oh that's a shame', or 'She's missed out' or 'I'm glad that I'm not in that situation, I'm happy that I've got my kids, or I've got my whatever'. I think that's probably the majority view, unless someone's been outwardly saying 'I don't want children', in which case they're either accepted or they're the next category, which I think is smaller, 'This person's selfish, she's not maternal, there's something wrong with her, she's unnatural.'

And this isn't just a modern phenomenon – Françoise, who is now in her 70s and was brought up as a Catholic, tried unsuccessfully to have children almost 50 years ago:

I think several people thought that I probably used birth control. I wasn't going to discuss my private life with them, so I didn't, because I was really quite successful in my career. So they thought it was my choice. I had some very hard things said to me – 'You'll regret it one day', 'You're just being selfish', 'Just because you're having a lovely time being a journalist…'

We (Rachel and Louise) have both been very successful in our chosen careers, and we have lost count of the number of times that other people have assumed that we have chosen to be childless (and that's just the ones that we're aware of!).

Helen sums up the irritation that many of us feel at being labelled in this way:

It really irritates me when people make assumptions about you – just because you're not having children, and you've got a really good job, they think that's all you care about, that you're just a career girl, and you get labelled as that. I think that's really unfair. I just hate that label, because there are all kinds of things that go with it. It's a negative label, you're a career woman, you selfishly want to pursue your own career, and are not interested in children, or having a family.

I really dislike that intensely – yes, I've got a good job, and I've done very well at work, but not because I chose to do that versus have a family. They just assume that means you're some kind of fairly hard-nosed, masculine-type person – it's OK for men to have successful careers, but I think it's less OK for women to have successful careers, unless you've got children as well, and you've juggled the whole lot, then you're truly superhuman.

Effects on our relationships with others

Not all of us face particular expectations from, or assumptions by, other people. However, as childless women, the majority of us do find that our relationships with members of our family and our friends are adversely affected in some way.

Kathryn, who talked about her experience of feeling either pitied or judged by other people, talks here about her relationship with her two sisters, both of whom are married with children:

I have a good relationship with both my sisters, but because they both have children I'll find that they socialise together a lot more, which is usually children based, in that the cousins want to. I understand that but occasionally, if I'm feeling a bit left out, it may feel that I'm actually a second-class citizen, which is not what they think at all, but sometimes it feels like that.

Occasionally, one of my sisters says to me, 'You're lucky, you've managed to go away on holiday', and I have to bite my tongue not to say 'I would actually swap with you, with what you've got'. Initially, I got annoyed when both of them were saying things like that, it felt like you're being selfish and we're being dutiful and having children. It felt unsympathetic, they knew what my feelings were, they didn't do it to hurt me, but they weren't thinking about it.

For Heather, getting divorced when she was in her mid-30s marked the start of having to face up to the possibility of not being a mother, which then became a certainty when she experienced an early menopause at 40. Her divorce also led to a radical change in her relationship with her sister and her nephews:

My older sister had two boys who I absolutely adored and who adored me. They would come and stay and everything else when they were young. My relationship with my sister, which is not what this is about, was very difficult, and when I actually split up from my husband, up until that stage we were legal guardians for the boys. She then wrote me this fairly horrendous letter saying because you're divorced you're no longer a suitable person so I'm going to hand over guardianship to somebody else. Which, again, took away, if you like, the only children I was ever likely to have. Not that I would have wanted them, because of the circumstances under which I would have got them...

The younger one, three years ago, committed suicide, which was horrendous for all of us, except I felt completely excluded by my sister, who kept saying, 'No one can understand anything like a mother's love.' If anything hurt me, that did. Because it's one of those things: you can't have children, and you deal with that, and then you're not even allowed to feel a love, that's denied to you as well. The whole thing then stirred up all sorts of stuff about not having children, so that was quite hard.

Helen, who shared her frustration at being labelled a 'career girl', talks here about her relationship with her mother, and her feeling of being isolated:

I personally haven't had lots of overt pressure, but I do feel as if I've found it harder to relate to my mum by not having children, and that she's found it harder to relate to me. My mum is a very traditional mum, she's got four children, her life has been very child centred, very much about the children, very much about her grandchildren; she's never worked outside the home. So in many ways we don't share a lot in common, in the sense of the route that our lives have gone, and sometimes I do think she finds it hard to relate to me, to have a relationship with me.

It's almost like the relationship that she has with my sister is a lot to do with children – her children, my sister's children – whereas with me it's like she can't really relate to my work ... it's almost like we don't have very much in common. I'm sad about it; it's back to this feeling isolated, back to not feeling that you can truly communicate with somebody else, that you truly understand one another.

This feeling of loneliness and isolation can be particularly strong if all around you, your friends are having babies and becoming engrossed in the demands of babyhood.

Sally married in her early 30s, and spent the first seven years of her marriage unsuccessfully trying to have a child:

When my friends were falling pregnant and having babies and their children were really tiny was definitely the worst time. When my friends stopped getting pregnant things felt a lot better. Having friends and family with kids who are 10 and upwards now feels fine, it's really nice.

Also when their children are very small, friends are very focused on them, they have to be, and if you don't have small children your life is so different from theirs you actually find that your friendship suffers. You're in one category, they're in another, they do different kind of holidays, they socialise with [other parents], so it puts you apart from your friends. There was a while when I felt quite separate and in a different category because I just didn't share this thing with my friends who had babies and children of the same age. That difference has actually disappeared now that their children are a bit older, the very small toddler/baby thing, it's a real bond between mothers, that's what they want to talk about. You're just not part of it.

All of that I found really quite hard, a lot of it is quite sad, you just think you don't share the same things – I just wanted to be like everybody else, I didn't want to be different.

What did surprise me was that, another friend who's a bit younger than me, she had a child about five years ago, and even when that happened, I found that really hard. You think 'Gosh, it actually hasn't gone away, it's just that people have stopped having babies so it feels better', but then when somebody did fall pregnant, the whole thing came back again.

Other people's pregnancies

While our childlessness can affect the nature of our relationships with members of our family and our friends, it can be their pregnancies that are particularly challenging and often very painful for us to deal with.

Kathryn, who talked about her relationship with her two sisters, both of whom have children, here talks about her feelings on hearing that the first of them was pregnant:

Then the next thing that happened was that my sister got pregnant. I just remember feeling awful about it, in that I couldn't be happy for her at the time. I tried to be, but I remember being so, so upset.

While the news of a pregnancy for someone close to you often prompts sadness, it may also lead to anger. Habie talked earlier about how total childlessness is never covered in the media. Here she reflects on her feelings about a friend's pregnancy:

We have a friend who doesn't like children. She doesn't hate them, because she's a nice human being, she likes people, but she has no interest in them whatsoever. Her partner is obsessed with children, so she said 'OK, I'm going to give you one month, one month off the pill, and if I'm not pregnant in one month, we're not having kids.' Of course she did get pregnant, and she had a little boy and he's lovely. She treats him like a little stranger in her home, someone you have to feed and you have to kiss and so on ... within three days of his birth, she brought him to meet us, and talked 100 per cent of the time about her work. The only thing she said about the birth that she'd had three days before was that she had this alien coming out of her body.

Her husband adores him and looks after him, and she's a very conscientious mother. But it really pisses me off to see that it's possible to not have this maternal instinct and still have children, and that Nature, Mother Nature, God, whoever it is, decided that I wouldn't, is just really horrible, unfair, disgusting, just makes me think that Mother Nature is a really bad mother. Because why give us the desire if we can't have the reality? It's like a design fault. Why make a maternal instinct and then create eggs that don't work after the age of 35 in some women?

It can be particularly difficult when you know that the pregnancy in question is unwanted. As Penny B, who talked about how religion helped her to cope with not being able to have a second child, says:

There was a lot of pressure, because many of my friends who'd had first babies with me were having their second babies, and I felt quite left out of the club. One really good friend had had her second child very unexpectedly and very soon after her first, and she was really not wanting the second child. So that was quite hard, listening to her saying 'Oh, I didn't want to get pregnant so soon', and there was me and this other friend saying, 'Oh, we just desperately want to be pregnant'. So nobody ever seemed to quite get what they wanted in the little club.

Marti, who is in her late 40s, has spent the last ten years since she married hoping to have a child, but has now accepted that it is unlikely to happen. For her, the pregnancy of other women in a similar situation can prompt feelings of both hope and jealousy.

I know two women who got pregnant at 44, both of them for the first time. They just kind of went to the doctor and said 'I'm putting on weight and I'm really tired', and the doctor says 'You're pregnant', and they both said 'What?' It's quite funny. So you kind of think maybe I'll be one of those. That's why you devour things like case histories in *Baby Hunger*, or whatever, because you think maybe there will be somebody else like me, that I can realise I'm not on my own, going through all this.

I do get jealous. I meet people, and I think 'Oh, she's as bad as me, she hasn't had children', and the next thing I know, she's having a baby, and I'm thinking 'That's not fair, how did she do that?' And I think about asking her, 'How did you do that, what have you been doing?', and then I think no. So I do get jealous of other people, particularly my peers who I thought were also in a similar situation to me, either because they haven't got married, or they haven't got pregnant or whatever else, and then they somehow manage to pull it off, and I think 'Shit!'

But it's also worth remembering that jealousy between childless women and women who are mothers is not all one-sided. Mary is in her late 60s, and celebrates her golden wedding this year.

My husband's eldest sister had three boys, and they really struggled because they had to bring three boys up. We were the first ones in the family to buy a house, and she was very jealous. She was also very jealous of all the clothes I bought and jealous of the holidays we went on. That made me very angry, because she'd got three things I wanted and I wasn't jealous of her. She couldn't see that if we'd had children, we wouldn't be doing all of these things.

How the news of a friend's pregnancy is broken can have a huge impact on the way we feel about it. Lucy B is unable to have her own children after having both ovaries removed:

It was extremely difficult, with one particular friend. I'd told her about my operation, before I went in, and she said 'I know everything's going to be all right'. Then afterwards, she phoned me and we spoke about it. She said how sorry she was, the usual sort of thing.

Then it was half-term week, my nephews were staying, my husband had just trotted off to work, and the post came. It was a notelet, and because it was the millennium and she'd been going to have a party I thought it was going to be a party invitation. I opened it up and it said 'I'm pregnant, we're having a baby'. I couldn't believe that she hadn't told me over the phone, or dealt with it in some better way than actually writing me this little note. My poor nephews were there, and I thought I don't want to go hysterical, which was exactly what I wanted to do, in front of them.

I was terribly hurt by that, and couldn't bring myself to speak to her properly for quite a while. I was just so hurt that she didn't have the strength of character to tell me herself, and deal with me being upset. That was what hurt me the most. The other thing that I didn't like, it was my first feeling of isolation, because I knew that everybody else would have known, and they would all have been discussing how the news was going to be broken to me.

Contrast Lucy B's experience with that of Sue:

My best friend's got three children. Every time she was pregnant, as soon as she could, even before she was through the danger time, she would tell me, because she didn't want me to find out from anyone else. She wanted to be the one to tell me, because she knew how much I wanted children and she wanted to be the one to break it to me as sensitively as possible. I respected her honesty and her thoughtfulness. And her courage – she didn't just phone me, she would come and see me. The first couple of times we were living about 30 miles from each other, but she would drive down to see me. I always knew, as soon as I opened the front door...

Inappropriate advice and platitudes

If we are prepared to tell other people of our unfulfilled desire for children, very often, what we get back is not the support and comfort that we were seeking, but advice (often inappropriate or unnecessary) or rather flippant comments that can feel very unsympathetic.

I (Rachel) desperately wanted to discuss my situation with good girlfriends, something I always did whenever I had a problem. I broached the subject with a handful of my best friends, but I didn't receive the kind of sympathy and support I craved. Those with children found it incredibly painful to hear my story. I think they felt powerless to help and very uncomfortable, even guilty that they had what I so desperately wanted. This usually resulted in 'Oh, you poor thing ...', followed by a desire to change the subject. A couple of chums incited me to cheat with contraception, revealing in minute detail how they had contrived their own 'mistakes'. In contrast, two childless friends of mine claimed they had never seen the appeal in having kids. Such responses only increased my sense of loneliness and isolation.

Incitements to cheat, or have an accident, are very common. Habie, who talked of her anger that it is possible not to have a maternal instinct and still have children, describes the situation when she was in a relationship in her 30s with a partner who had children from a previous relationship, and didn't want any more:

My friends were advising me to cheat, to have a baby behind his back, and I thought that's not fair, that's not fair on a man or on a child, to say 'Well, he never wanted to be your dad, but you're so pretty, he likes you now.' I mean, that's just wrong, so I never did it.

And when Clare A told her mother of her husband's infertility, her mother's advice was to chat up the milkman!

If the problem is that we are having difficulty getting pregnant, then we may well be faced with a list of things that we could try (as if women with fertility problems weren't already experts on the subject, having already devoured everything available in print and on the internet). Sally, who talked about feeling isolated and excluded when all her friends were having babies, was given all kinds of unhelpful advice:

People are well meaning, but before the problem was diagnosed you got friends and relations making a lot of well-meaning comments about changing your diet, or having sex in a different way, after sex lying with your legs on the wall. So what they're really saying is that it's your fault, as if you were having sex differently, more often, hanging your feet from the ceiling, eating differently, not smoking you would actually fall pregnant, and you begin to think it yourself. Because I had a fairly responsible job, people would be saying, even my husband was saying, 'It's stress, maybe you should take some time off work.' But I was perfectly happy at work, not stressed, if I took time off work I'd be really stressed, because I'd be doing nothing but waiting to become pregnant, and that's stress. It makes it seem like somehow it's your fault.

Natasha talked about the additional pressures of being Jewish, and here she shares the story of some unhelpful advice given to her at a dinner party:

I sat next to a really orthodox Jewish girl. We had a general conversation; then she said she had three children, and what did I have? 'One.' 'Oh, only one?' And I did my usual, and she pressed, 'Why have you only got one child?' I said 'Well actually, I can't have any more, I've been trying for years.'

She said to me, 'We were meant to sit next to each other, I have the answer for you. You have to come with me to the mikveh', which is a ritual Jewish bathing thing that you can do before you get married, and really orthodox Jewish women do it after their period every month and it's like a cleansing thing. I never did it at all. She said 'You need to come to the mikveh, to get rid of all your impurities.'

We ended up having this very civil but heated conversation at this dinner party. She really, really believed that it was because I wasn't a good Jew and that I hadn't been to the mikveh to get rid of all my impurities, that's why I wasn't getting pregnant, and that it was all within my control, I was not being a good religious soul and that's why I wasn't able to get pregnant. That was bizarre. I enjoyed the debate, because I'm that kind of person. She was lucky, because I wasn't offended. She could have so offended someone, by saying that to the wrong person, or hurt someone, seriously upset someone by her religious clap trap, really.

If we do tell people that we would like (or would have liked) children, one of the most common responses is 'you don't know how lucky you are'. Fay, who talked about how it can feel as though the whole of society is geared towards families, shares her frustration:

[One of the things that doesn't help] is people telling you that it isn't all a bed of roses to have children, that it's hard work. All the stuff they give you is absolutely true but doesn't help you at the time, because actually that's what you passionately wanted, you passionately wanted that experience. I can remember feeling like saying 'Sod that, I wanted it, warts and all'. Whether I would have liked it was another thing, but you know, you don't like it all, but I wanted it, and I didn't have that choice.

And a variation on this, of course, is 'you can always borrow mine'. I (Rachel) remember telling my brother how awful I felt about not having children and how lucky he was having such wonderful ones.

(He has a son through adoption and triplet daughters through IVF, whom he absolutely adores.) He jokingly replied 'Oh you're welcome to borrow mine, any time you like!' He didn't mean to upset me, but his flippancy really hurt me, it felt such a denial of my pain.

Thoughtless behaviours

Because many of us don't talk about the pain of childlessness, we may also have to face a range of thoughtless behaviours by other people. Sarah A, who found herself unexpectedly pregnant and then had a miscarriage a few days later, talks here about two incidents that were very painful for her:

About six weeks ago, a woman in the office, one of our administrators, came up to me and said 'Sarah, I have to show you this', and it was her scan photograph. That was such a shock, I thought 'Why would you do that?', and then I thought because it hasn't occurred to her that it's something that would be hurtful to me. And I thought why would anyone think it's something that would be hurtful to me? They obviously don't interpret me as being somebody who's coldly, clinically decided against having children, but I don't know what they do think.

It's the unexpected children that I find difficult, or the ones that weren't there, or weren't part of my life before I had this shock [the miscarriage]. A girlfriend who gave birth about April or May last year, who bombarded me with 'Oh, Sophie says thank you so much for the card' and then 'Please come and visit me', and I'm getting text messages from a 2-week-old baby, and this is very difficult.

I had to respond with 'I'm very sorry, but this isn't a good time for me at the moment. Happy baby talk is a little bit too distressing.' My friend immediately picked it up, but I was a little bit surprised – perhaps I'd never given off any vibes that this was a problem in my life before, and the last thing I was going to do was to tell her that I was pregnant, and then tell her that I'd had a miscarriage while she was actually pregnant. So that's actually ruined a friendship, because I have since not found the courage to pick up the phone and say 'Can I come and see you?', and the little girl's nearly one.

Penny talked earlier about the difficulty of coping with other people's second pregnancies, particularly where they weren't planned or wanted, and here she talks about the insensitive jokes that can be made:

I remember a plumber whose mate used to live next door to us. On Mothering Sunday, which I always find really hard, I walked into the park with a friend of ours, and he was there, and he said 'How many have you got?' I said one, and he said 'Haven't you managed the next one yet?' He thought he was being really funny, 'I'll have to tell your husband how to do it', and all this sort of stuff, and it really, really upset me. I can remember running home and bursting into tears, I was terribly uptight.

We can't really win either way – whether it's friends who are mothers telling us that we can't really understand what it's like because we haven't been through it, or childless friends telling us that they're really happy not to have children, it's difficult not to feel that we are being judged as inadequate, or having our pain denied.

Other emotional triggers

It may not only be the actions that are specifically directed at us by other people that unwittingly cause us pain, but also any behaviours or actions that reinforce our own sense of loss. My (Rachel's) particular pet hates are Christmas round robin letters in which everyone's child is a budding brain surgeon or flautist or both, and 'Baby on Board' car stickers. I detest them, but I know that in part it's because I've been denied the opportunities to use them myself.

Feeling angry about things that reinforce our sense of loss is not uncommon, as Lara's experience illustrates:

About three years ago, a neighbour of mine who is very artistic and had had four children of her own adopted a Chinese baby. I was so angry, my reaction, I was absolutely outraged, because she's getting on for 60. I was indignant. I think I was indignant because I wanted to say what the bloody hell do you think you're doing bringing up a little Chinese child, all on your own, and when you're dead, your children will have to look after that child. You've had four of your own ... I couldn't help it, I was absolutely enraged.

Like most of the women we talked to, Maria has, at times, felt excluded by the rest of the world:

All through my 30s, it was at the back of my mind. I just suddenly arrived in the age where everybody apart from me, it would appear, had children. And then you realise that people younger than you, when your friends are ten years younger are saying 'We're having a baby', and you think 'God, I'm miles behind you lot'. So you feel socially different, so that you're confronted with it. It's not really just the body clock, or whatever that biological hormone thing is, it's not just that, it's also the social thing. I just see that I'm a bit out of step with most of my peers who have done the husband, baby thing – some of my friends, their kids are teenagers. They could be grandmothers, my friends now.

It has taken Lucy A a long time to get over her feelings of being excluded:

Meanwhile of course all your friends are having babies, and you get ostracised because you don't have a child. They're off doing their little birthday parties, having their friends around where there's children and everything, and of course you have nothing to offer, so you don't get invited. They end up feeling embarrassed, in a way, and then you become isolated, through their embarrassment. They don't think you should be included, or don't know how to include you, or think it's something you wouldn't want, whereas in fact you'd be only too happy to be involved.

Childlessness – the taboo

The fact that there is a taboo, and childlessness isn't commonly talked about, undoubtedly makes our lives more difficult. So why does this taboo exist?

Often it can be easier to let other people assume that we're OK with our childlessness by putting a brave face on things. Elizabeth is in her mid-30s, and had to have a hysterectomy when she was barely out of her teens:

I find it quite difficult to verbalise. I suppose I just used to have this little sadness inside of me that just used to chip away. I probably never talked to anyone about it, I don't think anyone ever realised that actually this was something that I really wanted. I'm sure it works the same way for you – you're a career woman, you're in control, you're very articulate and intelligent, and you seem very sorted, so people just look at you and say 'Well, OK, you can't have kids, but you're clearly fine with it.'

Kathryn, who talked about her relationship with her sisters who are both married with children, talks here about her relationship with other childless/childfree friends:

I think that I've never had a completely honest conversation on both sides with any of my friends in that situation. I think there's a little bit of me that just doesn't want to say to anyone, 'Well actually this has been a really big deal for me, and it's been really upsetting.' I think it's been the same thing for them as well, there's been a little bit of keeping up appearances on all sides.

As well as wanting to protect ourselves, it can feel as though there is never an appropriate time to raise the issue. Rebecca B has never asked why her brother and his wife don't have children:

I'm never quite sure what the situation is but I think his wife biologically can't have children. Anyway, they're clearly not going to have any by now, I think, she's several years older than me. It would be interesting to talk to her about it, to see how she feels about it. I've never been completely sure whether it's that she can't have children or whether she just doesn't want to, and that's the kind of thing that, unless you just happen to be in the right kind of context, it is quite difficult to just ask somebody straight off. I don't know why that should be.

Lara makes the point that because our childlessness is ongoing, it may never feel like the right time to discuss it:

The way people live these days, there are always crises around that people are trying to manage. In the past it was much easier to chat about nothing, maybe because we were younger, and we could, whereas nowadays it's like whose parent is more ill than the other, whose is more demented than the other, whose daughter is coping with university or not, or on drugs, and somehow ordinary things like, but I'm still childless, are really beside the point. It isn't a crisis.

Lara also goes on to say:

I think anything that is different from the norm becomes taboo. It is normal for women to procreate, that's what they're built for, and we call that the norm. So I think that anything that veers away from the norm is a bit taboo.

As well as protecting ourselves, and not finding the right time to raise childlessness as an issue, we may also find ourselves wanting to protect other people by not talking about it.

Despite being very close to her mother, Linda never told her that she would have wanted more children:

My mother, my sister, other family members used to ask all the time. Why? And I just said, that was it, I've had enough and one was enough. I did tell my sister actually, but not anybody else, I never told my mother. I think because I didn't want her to be unhappy, I didn't want her to feel disappointed. I was absolutely sure that it would make her unhappy, and I could never, ever contribute to anything that would make her unhappy. It was part of, I suppose, being a good daughter, not doing anything wrong. I think I knew at the time she would have been a good support, but I definitely didn't want to disappoint her, and didn't want to burden her, and didn't want her to be unhappy.

Sally didn't want to embarrass other people:

You want to speak out because you just want to put a stop to gossip or speculation, and say 'This is me, this is my story', and I wonder why we don't do it. Sometimes I'm tempted at work, but then I think I would embarrass people. I just think if I say 'Well we always wanted children but we can't have them', I'm embarrassing them with too much information, I'm seeking sympathy or some kind of reaction, why have I placed that information in the public domain, it's for some kind of response or effect, and therefore you don't say it.

It is ten years since Anne B gave birth to a very premature son who lived for less than a day, and she would still like to be able to talk more about her experience:

The other big thing for me, when I lost the baby, was everybody's so sorry, everybody's really sorry, genuinely sorry, of course they are, but how long do you keep on talking about it? So I came to the conclusion that everybody has their ideal about how long they should be sorry about your loss. Then there's this cut-off point. When they reach that point, they cut off and then you don't talk about it any more. They decide I don't want to talk about it. They decide; enough's enough.

So there becomes this time when people don't want to talk about it any more, but I'd still want to talk about it. I'm not over it. You might be over it, but I'm not. You don't want to bore people, you don't want to be boring, but you're not over it, you want to talk about it. I'm not ashamed that I've had a baby. Of course I want to talk about it.

Why does everybody think we don't want to talk about it, when we do want to talk about it? Why is it a taboo subject? For what percentage of childless women is it a taboo subject, not to talk about it? I'd be really interested to know the answer, because I think everyone thinks that people don't want to talk about it, and I don't know, it certainly isn't the case with me. Because I'll talk about it, even now, at every opportunity.

Even women's magazines, which pride themselves on covering everything of importance in women's lives (and much that isn't), avoid childlessness. I (Rachel) remember feeling compelled to contact one editor after reading yet another article on the misery of miscarriage and the joys of longed-for children. I received a polite reply stating that if they ever decided to cover childlessness, they would invite my views. I wasn't asking for front page coverage, just an occasional acknowledgement of the existence of involuntary childlessness, and the grief it can bring. I'm still waiting.

But the rest of the world can help ...

From reading this chapter, it may feel as though our relationships with friends, families, work colleagues and acquaintances are inevitably going to be damaged by the fact that we remain childless, and that we are doomed to feeling excluded and isolated. However, it's not all doom and gloom – there are ways in which the rest of the world can help.

Friends and family can help, by giving us the opportunity to get involved with their children. While some childless women may not want to build relationships with children, finding it too painful, many of the women we talked to would have liked the chance to be more involved, but didn't feel that they were given that opportunity. Anne A knew from the age of 18 that she would not be able to have children of her own. She is grateful for the opportunities she was given to build relationships with her friends' children:

My friends were very kind, because they always let me make a fuss of their children. I've got friends, I used to take their boys for a walk, go over and take them in the pram. I had that, I suppose. It was a comfort. They all call me Aunty Anne, which is nice. It just makes me feel good, that they think that I'm worth calling Aunty Anne. I've got two godsons, one is now 31 and the other one is now 27. They come and see me and give me a big hug. They still make a fuss of me, which is very nice.

Several of the women we spoke to, such as Penny A, talked about how older women friends can help, often by giving us a sense of perspective:

My closest friend and I play the piano together once a week. She's 75 and she has two children, I'm really like a child, in terms of age, to her. I remember talking to her about it once and she said 'It's just a short stage of your life really, they grow up.' That really put it into perspective for me, I thought 'Yes, that's true.' If I had had children, aged 20, they would now have left home, and I wouldn't be so different in the way I live my life to now.

And finally, friends and family can be there for us just by listening, however uncomfortable that may be, without trying to tell us how lucky we are. All we need may be a glass of wine or a cup of coffee, and a hug, and someone to listen, without judging, advising us or trying to change the subject.

As Dr Rachel Naomi Remen says, in her book *Kitchen Table Wisdom: Stories That Heal*:

> *I suspect that the most basic and powerful way to connect to another person is to listen. Just listen. Perhaps the most important thing we ever give each other is our attention. And especially if it's given from the heart. When people are talking, there's no need to do anything but receive them. Just take them in. Listen to what they're saying. Care about it. Most times caring about it is even more important than understanding it. Most of us don't value ourselves or our love enough to know this. It has taken me a long time to believe in the power of simply saying 'I'm sorry' when someone is in pain. And meaning it.*

One of my patients told me that when she tried to tell her story people often interrupted to tell her that they once had something just like that happen to them. Subtly her pain became a story about themselves. Eventually she stopped talking to most people. It was just too lonely. We connect through listening. When we inter-rupt what someone is saying to let them know that we understand, we move the focus of attention to ourselves. When we listen, they know we care. (...)

I have even learned to respond to someone crying by just listening. In the old days I used to reach for the tissues, until I realised that passing a person a tissue may be just another way to shut them down, to take them out of their experience of sadness and grief. Now I just listen. When they have cried all they need to cry, they find me there with them.

This simple thing has not been that easy to learn. It certainly went against everything I had been taught since I was very young. I thought people listened only because they were too timid to speak or did not know the answer. A loving silence often has far more power to heal and to connect than the most well intentioned words.

Being childless will inevitably have an effect on our relationships with our family and friends. However, it doesn't necessarily have to damage them, as long as we can be honest about our feelings, and about what hurts us, and clear in what we need from other people – even if that's just someone to be with us and listen.

CHAPTER 7

Old age – fantasy and reality

Like many of the topics we discuss in this book, fears about old age are not something we'd really talked about before, either with each other or with our friends and families. We were therefore quite surprised that it turned out to be one of the most frequently recurring themes in our discussions with childless women. It seems to be an issue particularly for those of us who are single, and also for those of us in long-term relationships with an older partner who suspect, probably correctly, that we are likely to outlive our partners by a number of years.

In fact we discovered these fears are so common that they even have a name. Gail Sheehy, in her book *New Passages*, labels them 'Bag Lady Fears':

> *Women who have never married or spawned children have their own anxieties about the future. They may be worried about having no family members alive to look after them in their own old age. In fact, if one probes just beneath the calm, composed surfaces of the most successful and sophisticated middle-aged women – whether they be wedded, widowed, childless, or never married by choice – one is likely to find they have Bag Lady Fears. It was mildly astonishing to hear best-selling author Gloria Steinem, hit filmmaker Nora Ephron, superagent Joni Evans, former high-profile Planned Parenthood director Faye Wattleton,*

and many others (at the annual Power Lunch for Women at Manhattan's Rainbow room) admit that they have fears of finding themselves old, alone, forgotten or homeless.

What is it that we fear?

It can be quite difficult to probe beneath the surface of this fear, as for many of us it can be just too painful or scary to think about. We just try to ignore it and hope that it will go away.

A major part of the fear is definitely about being alone, and lonely, in old age. As childless women, feeling lonely and feeling excluded are things that we can suffer from at any age, but while we are still young enough and active enough we at least feel we can make an effort and do something about them. As we get older, this may well get more difficult.

Another major concern is the lack of any emotional and practical support that having children (and a partner) may provide. We all recognise that having children is no guarantee of having support in old age. Many of us even say that we would not have wanted the children we haven't had to be looking after us in old age out of a sense of duty. However, we do recognise that we may well need support as we get older, and it can be frightening not knowing where this will come from. This is probably made worse by the fact that many of us do not live in close communities, or with our extended families around us.

Rebecca B would love to have children, but her partner, who is 11 years older than her, is very reluctant:

I think the thing that most frightens me, actually, is the thought of being old and not having anyone. Particularly with my partner being older than me.

The thought of myself older, without children, is something that I find scary. It's this idea of life going through stages. When you're bringing up children you're putting all the effort in and looking after them. Traditionally, anyway, when you got older, they looked after you.

Obviously that's changing as society changes, and I don't necessarily think that a child's role is to look after their parents, even when they're grown up and so on, but it still seems to me that you get to a stage in your life where your children, even if they're not looking after you in that sense, are giving something back to you.

I'm quite frightened of getting to that stage in my life and not having that. When maybe you're too old to look outside the family any more, and there isn't really any family there to support you.

Finally, for many of us baby boomers, independence and control have been important values, possibly valued even more highly than usual because we haven't had children. The prospect of losing our independence, and becoming dependent on, presumably, faceless professional carers, can leave us feeling powerless and very vulnerable.

What triggers this fear of old age?

For many of us, it is the awareness that our own parents are growing older and needing increased support from us that provides the initial trigger to consider our own old age. This may be a gradual realisation or a sudden, dramatic one, such as when a parent dies, or develops a life-threatening illness.

If we become aware of these fears in middle age then at least we have the opportunity to reflect on them in advance. We can perhaps make some changes to our lives now, which can help to address our concerns about our own old age.

If, for whatever reason, we haven't considered these fears in advance, then it seems that there are two major triggers that can bring us face to face with the reality, and these are retirement from work or the loss of our partner.

As childless women, many of us throw ourselves into our work as a way of providing meaning, identity and fulfilment in our lives, and as a way of feeling needed and valued. When we retire from full-time employment, we may then have to face up to the issues of meaning and value all over again, as well as the specific fears and concerns about our impending old age.

Jane A was given early retirement from her full-time job four years ago, and reflects on her childlessness:

It gets worse as you get older, in a funny sort of way, unless you've got pots of money and you can just go pootling around the world all the time. I do have good friends, but everybody has their own lives and I just feel I need something, for me, really, that I haven't got at the moment.

In a way, although it was pretty horrible at the time, what happened four years ago was the best thing, because I've now had to re-look at things and think, 'Well, I haven't got that now', so you find other things to do instead.

Women in long-term relationships that manage to survive the crisis of being childless often report that the relationship becomes stronger and deeper as a result. However, if this happens to the exclusion of other friendships and independent activities, then the loss of your partner can be particularly traumatic.

Françoise was a successful journalist for many years. She is an elegant woman in her mid-70s, although when you talk to her, she seems much younger. She was very happily married for 43 years, and would have liked to have children, but after two miscarriages the medical profession told her there was nothing they could do. Her husband died four years ago, and following his death she has moved to a new house in a different village:

It's now I miss children. Desperately.

I look at people who are grandmothers and I envy them, but what worries me now is my terrible loneliness. All my friends with children ... if I cry, please forgive me ... I'd like to have grandchildren, but I can't say I think about it a lot, it's the fact that I've got nobody to ring up. That's where I envy people with children, and children who take trouble about their parents. Not that one wants to get in the way. Maybe I'm wrong; maybe I'm seeing it in the wrong way.

Somebody was saying to me the other day, you know, 40, 50, 60 years ago older people lived with their children, or their nephews and nieces or their godchildren or something, because there was nowhere else. Now everybody goes into homes, or buys different houses and people live in different places. Maybe I'm fantasising, but at the moment I'm suffering terribly, not having children.

I feel very guilty about asking people for support, you know. I don't know whether people feel guilty about asking their children, or making it known to their children, I don't know. I don't usually ask. I'm never somebody who rings up and says 'Can I have coffee with you, I'm feeling miserable?'

At the moment, I haven't got an interesting life, and I don't really want to go on living an awfully long time. Honestly, what's the point? If you have children and grandchildren there is a point.

But for some women, such as Habie, the fear of being old and childless is not triggered by anything specific, but is ever present:

To be honest with you, the old maid on the shelf is a fear that I feel at least once a day, I worry about that. The thought of getting older, when my wrinkles come, and I have no children, then I get old, altogether old, and have no grandchildren, how will that be bearable? How is it possible to go through it twice, once as a mother and once as a grandmother, when all your friends are grandmothers, and all your siblings, and you aren't? Then how will I be a woman? How will I be an old lady with no descendants? That is just so scary I can't even think about it.

Our fears about old age are reinforced by the lack of any positive imagery of women in old age – other than as a matriarch, of course, surrounded by an ever expanding pyramid of several generations of family. When we think of single, childless, old women, we are more likely to think of someone slightly dotty, wandering the streets, talking to herself and feeding the pigeons, or stuck at home (or in a home) watching daytime TV, rather than any more positive role model to which to aspire.

Grandchildren – the ongoing loss

Our fears about old age may emerge when the first of our friends, or our siblings, or even, in some cases, our partner, becomes a grandparent. Not having grandchildren can be a double loss – not only do we miss out on the apparent 'pleasure without responsibility' that grandchildren seem to provide, but not having grandchildren may reinforce and rekindle our earlier loss in not having children of our own. This may be particularly difficult when friends and work colleagues are becoming grandparents in their 40s, at a stage in their lives when we are only just learning to accept and live with our own childlessness.

Heather discovered that she was menopausal in her late 30s, while she was trying to get pregnant. At the time she threw herself into her work as a way of coping, but recently, after 15 years, the issue resurfaced:

My nephew's partner had a baby at Christmas and I was suddenly faced with not only couldn't I have my own children, but I'd never have my own grandchildren. That hit me, and yes I should have expected it, but I didn't. I hadn't focused on it at all.

I couldn't actually go and see the baby for about five days. I couldn't actually do it. And interestingly enough it was my nephew's partner who called me and actually invited me over. Everyone else was dropping in, and she phoned me up and said 'It would be really lovely if you could come over for coffee.' I got there, and she said 'Are you finding it difficult?' It was so lovely of her, because of course once I'd seen the baby, I was fine. Because it was nothing to do with the baby at all, it was everything to do with me.

I guess what surprised me is I've gone through this range of really not being worried about not having children when I was married and I was younger, to suddenly these huge gaps that that creates. Gaps that will be there now for ever. If that makes any sense at all.

And grandmothers can be even more tactless and insensitive than mothers, when it comes to showing photographs and boasting about their grandchildren's achievements – as one woman said 'they just go off on to another planet, grandmother world'.

How to address the fears of old age

Many of the strategies for learning to live with childlessness, in terms of alternative ways of finding meaning and value and of making a contribution, are applicable at any age.

But one of the things that we can do to prepare for old age specifically, is to think about it now, rather than ignoring it and hoping it will go away. When I (Louise) first experienced this fear, I thought it was a sign of weakness. I felt rather ashamed, and tried to pretend it hadn't happened. Now, I am very reassured to realise that I am by no means alone in having these fears, and that there are things I can do now to address them.

For me, it has been important to face the fear, and consider which particular aspects of the bag lady fantasy concern me the most. The sorts of questions I have been asking myself include: Is the place where I live now a place in which I can imagine growing old? Do I have a strong network of family and friends (other than a partner) locally? Do I have good relationships with my neighbours, and in the wider local community? If you ask yourself these questions, and answer 'No' to any of them, what could you do about it?

Looking at the most extreme solution, moving house and building a new life in a completely different area is much easier in your 40s or 50s than it is in your 70s ... Even if you don't feel that you need to go that far, then there may be changes that you want to make now to your lifestyle and activities that will help ease the transition later on.

As a result of unexplained infertility, Mary and her husband have no children. When he retired about ten years ago they moved out of the city into a small, rural community.

My husband joined the golf club, I joined the sewing club, we joined the gardening club, we joined the history club. We weren't joiners before we moved here, funnily enough, we've never joined clubs before, but I thought it was important that we developed a social life for later in life.

You all need people to help you later on, and I found in the city you just didn't make that sort of friendship with neighbours. I think neighbours become the important people in your life when you get old, more so than family. Someone could come and help you within half-an-hour here, do something for you that would only take half-an-hour out of their daytime, whereas a member of the family you've got to phone, they have an hour-and-a-half's drive, you couldn't do that if you wanted a pint of milk up the road, could you?

So everybody here, it's a wonderful little set up, even though we call it God's waiting room because most are elderly, but we'll all help each other in a crisis, and I think at this stage in our life, that's important.

And what about the children whom you do have in your life? We all have them – nephews and nieces, godchildren, friends' children – how do you feel about your relationships with them now, and how would you like to see these relationships develop, as you (and they) grow older? Perhaps this is a solution to those insensitive grandmothers – we could carry photos of our nephews and nieces, godchildren – or even our pets!

For Marti, like a number of women we talked to, drawing up her will has helped her to feel more prepared for childless old age:

I've done my will, and he (my husband) gets some, and they (my nephews and nieces) get lots. So I feel I'm helping them out, and able to think 'OK, so I can't have my own children and look after them, but I can at least make sure that they (my nephews and nieces) can put a deposit on a flat or do whatever when they grow up.'

It's also worth reflecting that being a grandmother, as with being a mother, can often appear more attractive from the 'outside' than it does from the 'inside' – there is a danger that we look at it through rose-tinted glasses. It is estimated that the childcare provided by grandparents is worth £1 billion per year in the UK, with the number of children being cared for by grandparents at least part of the time having increased from 33 per cent to 82 per cent over the last two generations. There is a similar picture around the world: the latest census figures for New Zealand, for example, show over 4000 grandparents had taken on the role of parent to their grand-children. Pleasure without responsibility appears to be a myth for the grandmothers of today; in New Zealand, there are now 26 support groups around the country for grandparents raising grand-children, and in the UK there is even an action group, Grandparents Plus, which was set up to lobby for the rights of grandparents.

Old age – rewriting the rules

Our fears of old age may be widespread, if unspoken, but that is no reason to assume that they will inevitably come to pass. We've lived the first 40 (or 50, or 60) years of our lives in a very different way from our mothers' generation – why shouldn't the last 20 or 30 years be different too?

As baby boomers, we are noted for rewriting the rules. There's no reason why childless old age shouldn't be a liberating, rather than a depressing, experience. No children to support financially through further education and getting them on to the housing ladder; no grandchildren to provide unpaid care for; no concerns about looking after heirlooms for the next generation – I (Rachel) happily put our gold-leaf dinner service in the dishwasher, against all the manufacturer's advice, and Douglas and I joke about dying leaving the biggest overdraft in history, a fantasy shared by other childless women we have spoken to!

Although not specifically for childless women, the Red Hat Society (see Appendix 1) is a great example of women rewriting the rules. The society is a fast-growing movement of women who are finding a new way to embrace, and even celebrate, the ageing process. Founding member Sue Ellen Cooper was inspired by the poem *Warning*, written by Jenny Joseph in 1961, which opens:

> *When I am an old woman I shall wear purple*
> *With a red hat which doesn't go, and doesn't suit me*

Membership is open to all women, but only those aged 50 and over can wear the official attire of the club – red hats and purple outfits. And, as Sarah A says:

I'm sure we'll have great coping mechanisms, because there will be all these feisty women who'll make it work, these retirement communities that people move into in their 50s, with golf course, swimming pool, health club, spa etc., etc. There'll be a few more handrails, but we'll all be doing morning aerobics so we won't be seizing up so much.

CHAPTER 8
Coping mechanisms

None of us can escape the reality of stress and pain in our lives, and we all have different ways of coping. We may favour one particular mechanism, or we may use a variety of methods – work, displacement activity, rationalisation, food, drink, denial – the list is long.

Faced with the stress and the pain of wanting a child and not having one, our coping mechanisms are essentially reactive – they are a response to the pain of our childlessness, which allow us to avoid its intensity until, over time, that intensity eventually fades. When that happens, we can either choose to live with the pain – ignoring it most of the time apart from an occasional pang – or perhaps we can begin to face our childlessness and explore it.

Although coping mechanisms have an important role to play, they can become excessive or even dysfunctional, in an attempt to block out the pain. Our coping mechanisms can become a habit, as we continue with the behaviours involved, even after the intensity of the pain we are dealing with has faded to a more manageable level and the purpose the coping mechanisms served has gone. It is therefore useful to review our coping mechanisms from time to time to ensure they are still appropriate.

Focusing on other things

One of the most common ways of avoiding pain is to distract ourselves in some way. For the baby boomer generation in particular, focusing our time and energy on work is very common. It can also help to restore our self-confidence and self-esteem by allowing us to find success and a sense of achievement at a time when our sense of self-worth may have been seriously undermined by our childlessness.

I (Rachel) had workaholic, perfectionist tendencies from an early age, so when faced with childlessness it was only natural to throw myself wholeheartedly into work. What's more, the power I wielded and the money I earned helped to anaesthetise the pain and gave me a sense of control, purpose and self-worth. I continued working all hours for over a decade, enjoying the success. Then one day, quite suddenly, I felt incredibly weary and realised that my overtly successful lifestyle was pretty dysfunctional, and that work was devouring me.

I can see now that had I turned to drink, drugs or food rather than work, I and others might well have spotted the problem far sooner. But in our society, a live to work philosophy is rewarded. The realisation that work had become a problem not the solution came in a flash, but what I do and who I am, if not a workaholic, is taking much longer to work out. I'm in uncharted waters. I suppose it's my identity that I'm trying to grapple with – if I'm not a mother, and I no longer find total fulfilment through work, then who am I? I realise that I need to construct my own identity, as society's options for middle-aged women look to be limited to mother, career woman or both.

Jane A is single, and has recently retired. She looks back at the time in her early 40s when she recognised that she was unlikely to have children:

I think it made work too important. I would sit at work, there was another friend at work who had a child when she was a bit older, and of course she'd just disappear at whatever time because she had to go and pick the little girl up, and there you are, sitting there doing goodness knows what, thinking what am I doing here? I think I would have put less emphasis on work if I'd had children, because you wouldn't have had the time, would you, you wouldn't have sat there until 8 at night, because you would have got home because you would have had something else to do. So it's the fact that work filled the gap, and it shouldn't have done, I know it shouldn't have done.

Sarah A has a game that she plays with herself to assess how well her distraction strategy of keeping busy is working:

I need to try and work this out, I want to get to a point where I wake up one morning and it isn't there. I almost have a little game, it's not quite a game, but it's how late in the day is it before you first remember that you can't have children, or that it's an issue? It comes back a lot, and I have coping strategies, and the best one is to be busy. If I'm really busy, and caught up with work, and caught up with social life, and caught up with friends, then days go past, but then there's another part of me that's horrified that I'm letting the days go past.

Work is not the only way in which we try to deflect or manage the pain. For Habie, it's about focusing on the things that can give you pleasure, even when you may not really feel like it:

I do believe that friends and the things that you enjoy in your life really do make a difference, because they stop you thinking about pain. They let you live your life, so I guess the things that I love are the cinema, even then it's lost a bit of its shine with all the pain, but I still love it, I love being in the garden with my partner, I love just being with him, and I love reading and telly and when I do those things it helps. But that's probably a bit of a wishy-washy answer, because it's just life, life helps. But there isn't a technique. But one thing I would say is, do not mope. Do not be alone at home without a job to do and still think you're going to get over your childlessness. Because then all you do is run around in circles, suffering. So if you force yourself in those times to go for a swim, or a walk, or go and see friends ... I think friends are essential.

Judy is in her late 40s. She and her husband are actively engaged in exploring overseas adoption, and have not ruled out the possibility of egg donation. Judy recognises that many aspects of her life are, on some level, substitution activity for not having her own family.

I'm really worried that on a bad day I can say that all of this is just displacement activity. Judy, you've just bought a new house, that's just displacement activity for getting on with the real issues. Why did you do that? Why did you disrupt your life and take on more financial responsibilities when you could be focusing in on having kids. Why did you take this stupid job? I think 'Wow, OK, well it's because you've got a crisis of self-confidence and you still need to prove something.'

Heather focuses her time and energy on voluntary work:

I look at people like my godson's parents and they have got something to show for their life. And I haven't. So then I do even more voluntary work, and I just run myself absolutely ragged, and everyone says 'Why are you doing it?', and I can't explain to them why I'm doing it. It's probably displacement activity, actually, and it's just transferring something.

Heather's dreams of children came to an abrupt end when she entered the menopause in her late 30s. Her immediate reaction was to take herself away from it all:

I did go away on holiday, I treated myself just to get away from all the situations that were going on around, something completely different. Running away, but with a purpose: the purpose was because I was at a physically low ebb, but getting better, a bit of sunshine and relaxation to help that process never hurt anyone. So I did that, and then I threw myself into work, and dealt with it that way. Which is what I've always done, over anything, so that's just the pattern.

Although not very good at it, I (Rachel) totally agree with the benefits of relaxation. I think being kind to yourself can help enormously. Over the last few years, I've got into the habit of treating myself to things like aromatherapy massages and reflexology sessions, which I find incredibly comforting. Sometimes, just buying glossy magazines or a lipstick does the trick.

It may sound a bit alternative, but I've also taken to going to a flotation centre. Lying in total darkness, suspended in warm water, sensory deprivation quickly leads to deep relaxation, freeing the mind to experience wonderfully weird, very vivid semi-conscious dreams, sensations and visions. During a recent float, my mind wandered and I found myself surrounded by identical little cherubs, and I realised that I was in Heaven! On closer examination, I recognised them from old photos of my husband as a child. Yet the way they were all so active and busy reminded me of myself. I suddenly realised they were our children, and they said 'Don't worry, Mum, we're much better off here, we're having a lovely life. If we'd been born, we'd have had loads of worries, exams, work, we're much better off here. You did us a favour, thanks.' It was a very bizarre experience, but one I found strangely comforting. It seemed to allow me to let go of some of the last vestiges of the angst I was harbouring around my childlessness, and has brought me a new sense of peace.

Another form that distraction can take is the use of humour to lighten the pain. I (Louise) used to joke that on my 40th birthday, I'd gone from being too young to have children to being too old to have children overnight!

Mary and her husband tried for many years to have children, and had various tests, but their infertility was ultimately unexplained. Mary jokes:

I can't remember when I stopped looking every 28 days and saying, 'Oh, that's another one.' You know, I could joke then 'That's my hundredth miscarriage I've just had.'

Even now, almost 50 years later, Mary and her husband still joke about it:

We joke about being grandparents, when we do go out to zoos and things like that, which we do, we do all the things that grandparents do, but we haven't got the grandchildren tagging behind us, crying for an ice cream.

But, as Eve says:

It's easy to be flippant about it as a way of avoiding feeling pain. It's easy to say to people, 'Well at least I don't have to do this for them, and I don't have to entertain them, ha, ha, ha.' I think it would have been quite easy to say that whilst deep down feeling 'But I wanted them.' I do feel now I can look back on it, or look at myself, and I can laugh about it sometimes. I can make a flippant joke about not having children and it doesn't bother me any more. It's a tinge of regret rather than a full-blown sadness, I suppose.

Rationalisation

Rationalisation can be another common way of not allowing ourselves to feel the pain, by reminding ourselves that there are things in our lives to feel good about or by telling ourselves that things could always be worse.

For Kathryn, who is single and in her early 40s, it's about now looking at her childlessness logically, rather than emotionally.

A couple of years ago I went through a stage of waking up every morning and thinking 37... 37. I've got to get pregnant soon or I'll never have a baby. It was just such a miserable situation, and I'm not like that any more, which is a relief.

At the moment, I guess I'm probably starting to come to terms with the fact logically that I'm not going to have children, and I'm not rushing myself too much about that. I think the fact that I'm thinking 'No, I'm not going to have children', means that I'm just worrying less about it, it just used to take up so much time and energy.

I'll probably need to continue with this logical way of thinking, rather than emotional thinking about it, so that I'm feeling less childless and less shamed, and less unfinished, and I can say to myself 'OK, that didn't happen, but I'm not the only person in the world it didn't happen to, I'm not any less of a person for it.' It's the logical sorting out, rather than being dragged down by it, being dragged along by my emotions.

Elaine's rationalisation takes the form of wondering whether, deep down, she actually wanted children or whether it was just social conditioning:

Sometimes I wonder whether I really, really wanted them, because not having them hasn't been as decimating to me as with some people I've seen. I haven't had the depths of despair, can't get out of bed, can't function, just that level of grief and been completely wiped out by it, I've not had that. I keep saying 'I didn't plan to be here, I never intended to be single and childless', but I wonder if maybe deep down inside, I subconsciously did, and whether I've gotten to where I want to be. But because it's such a no-no in society, I'd rather use the 'Well, I never met anybody, I've had loads of relationships and they've all failed, blah, blah, blah' as the excuse for being where I probably wanted to be anyway. Sometimes I think that's probably the reality.

But I know the constant thought, my last thought at night when I go to bed is 'I'm single and childless' and my first thought when I wake up in the morning is 'I'm a failure, I'm single, nobody loves me, I've got no kids, there's nothing' – the only constant emotional thing in my life apart from my friends is my cat. It's probably more upsetting than I'm allowing it to be.

Another common form of rationalisation is to remind ourselves of the downsides of having children.

Sarah A, who talked earlier about the game she plays to assess how successfully she is distracting herself, also helps out with her local Girl Guides:

There's joy about them, but they're also quite a good little reminder the other way, because they can be bloody annoying, and you think 'Yeah, mine could have turned out like that.'

Lucy A appreciates not having to deal with the guilt she sees associated with juggling being a mother and being a professional businesswoman:

A lot of my contemporaries have full-time jobs, and they're having to get au pairs and nannies. So it's 'Is the nanny the right nanny?', 'Am I going to see my children?', 'I've got a business meeting tonight, I haven't seen my kid for two days.' I'm glad I don't have to go through all that; I haven't got any of those guilt feelings.

Debbie recognises that, as a childless woman, she doesn't have all the worries that go with having children:

In an odd sort of way, I think I'm happier because I don't have to worry about a child, and of course I would. My mother is someone who can't have sharp pencils in the house in case a child falls on them and blinds themselves. I would never be that bad, but I would worry about things – you do.

Clare A also recognises the negative side of having children, particularly seeing the problems that some of her friends are now having with their teenage offspring. However, like many of the women we spoke to, she also talks about the positive aspects of not having children:

It's not all doom and gloom, I have had, materially, a very lucky life, have travelled a lot, can do just about anything I want really, in terms of having the freedom. So there are advantages too, but it's not something I would have chosen.

For Helen, focusing on the positives of what you do have is core to her philosophy:

I'd much rather focus on the really positive things that I have, and really learn to be content with what I do have, rather than be chasing what I don't have. That's really core to me, actually, that whole concept of accepting that you don't get everything that you want in life, nobody has a perfect life, nobody has absolutely everything they want, and you have to be really glad and happy and thankful for the good things that you have, and really enjoy them, and make the most of them.

I do think that not having children gives you opportunities that you don't have if you have children, and you have to work at it, I think. You know I work through all the positives, I am very happily married, I really enjoy being married to my husband, we have really good fun together. We have lots of friends, lots of family, lots of people, we do lots of things together, we are in an incredibly fortunate position to be able to have lots of fun, really. We travel quite a lot, we have people to stay, because this is a childfree zone, having people who've got children, they almost all love coming to stay with us, because it's not a child-friendly house.

Clare B was initially devastated when, after ten years of marriage, her husband said that he really didn't want children. However, as she started to consider the positives of remaining childless, her attitude changed:

It wasn't long that I was really upset before I started to think really hard about what it meant, and what it meant to me, what it would mean to my life, if I didn't have children. It was quite extraordinary; it was like suddenly there was a great weight lifted off my shoulders. It was really quite a physical feeling. I thought 'I will be free to do whatever I want to do.' It was just like suddenly getting that realisation. I suddenly thought 'Well I could quite enjoy that.' I thought about it over more time and stuff, and you know that felt right, I felt happy with that.

Trying to find a reason

For a number of the women we spoke to, one important coping mechanism was trying to work out why they had ended up childless, feeling that if they could find a specific reason for their childlessness, it would make it easier to cope with.

Mary, who joked about her losses earlier, thought she was going to 'inherit' children, through friends or family dying:

A dear friend suddenly rang up out of the blue and said 'I want to ask you something. If anything happened to my husband and I, we want to know that the children would be cared for. Would you look after the children, because we want to do it in writing somewhere, legally.' Without any hesitation, I said yes. Then I thought, 'God, I could end up with three kids, all growing up.' But I didn't hesitate.

Also, I went to a fortune teller once who told me I was going to have three sons. My husband's elder sister's got three boys, so for ages I thought they were going to get killed somewhere. I said to my husband, 'Would it follow that we'd have them?', and he said 'I suppose so.' For ages, I was waiting for them to have an accident.

Sally also spent time trying to find a reason for her childlessness:

I used to think there must be a reason that we haven't got children, and the reason might be, for the sake of argument, that my brother, my nieces and nephews are all growing up now, my brother and his wife would be killed in an air crash or something, and we'd have to look after their children. That would be the reason, and we'd be there to look after them. Or maybe that we would die very young, and we'd leave our children orphaned at a very young age, that's why, because that would be horrible as well, because there must be a reason, but of course there isn't a reason. You do try to search for a meaning in it, or some kind of logic, but it's not fair, and that's not how it is.

For Lesley, it's about wondering whether there was some deeper purpose to her remaining childless:

I do believe that things are as they are for some kind of purpose. So I ask why? It's not desperate grief or anything, it's why me, just why did it all work out like this? How have I ended up like this, and is there some deeper purpose to all of this? Is it that I do try and help other people? Maybe that's the answer, I don't know.

Avoiding children

For many childless women, when grief is raw, it may be necessary to avoid spending time with children because it's just too painful.

After Anne B had given birth to a very premature baby, who only lived for 24 hours, she found that, while she was fine spending time with the children who were already in her life, she just couldn't be around people with new babies:

My cousin had had a miscarriage, then she'd had a baby, the same time as I'd had mine. I couldn't have anything to do with her, or the child. Now as horrible as that might sound, I couldn't. I couldn't have anything to do with anyone who'd got a new baby. But if I'd known that child before, I had no problem with it.

Lucy B actually considered moving house to avoid being around babies, after having both ovaries removed when she was in her early 30s:

When we moved here, although we live opposite a playground there weren't many children in the houses. Then, it must have been the first summer after my operation, a family moved in over there with babies. I was lying in the garden, reading and relaxing, and heard this crying baby noise. I thought I'm going to have to tell my husband that we're going to have to move, because I can't bear if I'm surrounded by babies crying, and can't escape even in my home where I feel I should be safe from this.

Heather talked earlier about running herself ragged with voluntary work. When her dreams of having children first came to an abrupt end, she found it impossible to spend time around families:

I remember for the first two or three months, just walking around looking at families, thinking I can't do this. I looked at them and I couldn't go to anything where there were families. The guy I was then in a relationship with has two daughters. I was working in the States and he'd arranged to take them to Disneyworld in Florida, and I was going down to join them. I arrived in Orlando and I said 'I'll stay in the house with you, but I cannot come to Disneyworld.' I could not go. I just physically couldn't do it. I don't know what it was, whether it was jealousy or envy or whatever; it was just the most awful feeling.

Ultimately, as Rebecca A says, it is important that we are honest about what hurts us:

There are some new neighbours that have moved in down the road, and they have a little 11-month-old baby boy. She invited me to go to a picnic with her and the baby and other women and children, and I had to be very honest and say 'I can't do that, it would be too painful for me, because I will wish I had a child to take to it.' That was very honest, but it was much better for me to do that than to make some excuse, 'Oh I can't come, I'd love to but I can't come', because then she might have asked me again, and I'd go through that pain again.

As a teenager, I (Rachel) taught children to swim, and twice worked abroad as an au pair. I enjoyed being around children. However, while working on the book and hearing childless women talking so fondly about their relationships with children, I realised just how much I'd blocked children out of my life, since knowing that we wouldn't have any of our own.

I invariably give new mums gifts of soap or champagne, claiming they're probably snowed under with baby clothes. I've declined numerous requests to be a godmother on the grounds that I don't feel sufficiently religious. I set up baby bond savings schemes for my nephews and nieces, saying I wouldn't know what to buy them. If possible, I try to see friends who are mums in the evenings.

I'd isolated myself from children for the last 15 years, but I'd become so good at rationalising my decisions that I hadn't realised that what had been an initial necessity to cope with the pain of childlessness had become a way of life. I wanted to reconnect with children, but the idea terrified me, like opening up an old wound. However, no sooner had I mentally made that decision than my brother asked if I'd accompany him and his four children to Disneyworld, Florida. I was scared, but I agreed and we had a ball. By facing one of my worst fears, I'd been released from it, and had taken another step on my road to recovery.

Putting pain 'in a box'

In some ways, all of the above coping strategies can be seen as ways of avoiding feeling the pain of childlessness, or at least containing or segregating the pain, allowing us to get on with the rest of our lives in a reasonably functional way. Many of the women we interviewed openly acknowledged this.

For Liz and her partner it's about accepting their childlessness and getting on with life:

I think we've determined to put it (our childlessness) in a box, and just pop it up on a shelf and continue on with life. Every now and then there are things that prickle, I suppose, and it's usually a nice thing, and you think 'Gosh that's a pleasure I won't enjoy.' When you see a child in a very loving cuddle with a parent, when you see a child who's distressed and where their parents are helping them deal with a problem, you think 'Aah, that's nice, and I'll never have that.'

For Eve, it's about not dwelling on her childlessness:

It doesn't bother me nearly so much now, I think because I don't let myself think about it. It's a road that I just don't go down any more. I could really sit and think about it and dwell on it and I would get upset, but, as I said, I don't let myself go down that road, because I don't see any point in it.

And at the end of most of our interviews, we asked women to draw a picture to represent their childlessness – it's interesting how many of the pictures included boxes, sacks or frames.

While we were on the lookout for women to interview for this book, I (Rachel) spoke to two close girlfriends, both married and childless, with whom I can normally chat unreservedly about almost anything. On hearing about the project, both visibly froze. One said she had never really discussed her childlessness with anyone; it was just too painful to even think about, let alone discuss. It was as though she feared that to speak about her feelings would unleash an uncontrollable tidal wave of emotion, and she just couldn't take that risk. The subject was clearly intensely painful, even though it transpired that she has lived with the diagnosis of unexplained infertility for almost 20 years. The other girlfriend said nothing, and despite seeing her regularly, she has never once mentioned the book, so something that is intended to open up the subject has itself become a taboo.

As Alison Bagshawe, Senior Fertility Counsellor at Guy's Hospital, says, putting our experience in a box can be a good or a bad coping mechanism, depending on our feelings about what we have shut away:

Putting your experience in a box can be fine; it's how you feel about it. If you find that the lid is lifting up, or there's rattling in the box, whenever you see a baby, then it can be difficult. Everybody's make-up is different. For some it is much easier to box it up, that is their coping mechanism, it probably always has been, in which case it might well work for them. So there's no right or wrong way about this, but my guess is that it's protective. 'This is my secret box, my safe box, don't come into it, back off'. And that's fine if they really do feel safe in that box, that's fantastic, good for them, they've managed to do something that a lot of people can't. But if it's like a jack in the box, it's always wanting to get out, if it actually prevents them doing things with their lives like going to christenings, being godparents, doing things which might involve children, then most probably it will not be a comfortable box to be in.

And as Liz Scott, Fertility Counsellor at the Assisted Conception Unit of the Lister Hospital, says, ultimately, bottling up our experience can be self-destructive:

As women, we have a societal view that one doesn't display anger, so a lot of it gets internalised, and blame gets apportioned in different areas. But there's huge anger, because of the unfairness of it. Fertility is not distributed fairly, and there's a very cruel element to it as well. For example, you're working with someone and she's just had a still-birth, and her best friend phones up and tells her that she's pregnant, and she's struggling with these issues. Or someone at work is moaning about the fact that she's pregnant, because she forgot to take the pill, and there's such rage.

It's OK, but these are such primitive feelings that we operate with, which just tend to well up. Or we put them back in the bottle with the stopper on, and sometimes, at very inopportune moments, it all comes up and it can be very destructive. Sometimes we can turn it in on ourselves, as depression, very negative feelings, self-destructive feelings, lowering of self-esteem. Anger, jealousy: they're primitive survival skills; they're helping us to survive. Because we feel angry, it has the potential to move us on. But if we don't allow ourselves to be angry, we stuff it in and it takes other routes, and it can become self-destructive.

Coping mechanisms can be a useful tool to make living with the pain of childlessness bearable. Indeed, for some of us, the sorts of mechanisms we've talked about may be enough to enable us to learn to live with our childlessness. For others, while the coping mechanisms can provide a breathing space to deal with the initial intensity of the pain, it may then be necessary to work through the pain and grief of childlessness, with or without professional help, in order to be able to move on.

CHAPTER 9

Dealing with grief

The nature of grief

Wanting a child and not being able to have one, for whatever reason, can result in a whole multitude of different emotions, but grief differs from other emotions in a number of ways, which we need to recognise if we are to deal with our grief successfully.

First, whether we feel it as sadness, despair, disappointment or regret, all of us who are childless through circumstances rather than choice will experience grief in some form. Some of us may also feel angry, or guilty, or ashamed, but we will all feel sad.

And it's not simply the sadness of not having a child, but it's the loss of everything that child represents for us. It may include everything from wanting to be pregnant, give birth and breast feed, to having a stake in the future, passing on our values to the next generation, being 'normal' or part of a 'proper' family. The list goes on and on ... the loss is enormous and multifaceted.

Elisabeth is in her early 40s and single. Her father died when she was a small child, and her mother died when she was in her teens:

I've got a close friend who's almost exactly my age, she's very different to me, but she too has no partner or child, and we don't feel the same way. She is sad about not having had children, but not in a physical way. I don't think she would get tearful about it as I do, I mean I just have to think about it, walking down the road ... I think it represents a lot for me, I think it represents something to do with life force and this feeling of the woman I could have been and am not. Somehow the whole baby thing has got me in touch with sadness about a lot of things, I think.

Grief can be all-consuming, making it difficult if not impossible to even function normally. Habie has been desperately trying to have a child with her partner for seven years, including three failed pregnancies:

Every time I see a dark little girl, I think of Maia, our baby who we lost, or the other one, little Bean, who we also lost through miscarriage, I think that could have been her. If I see a child with intelligent, shining eyes, talking animatedly to their friends or their parents in a public place, I immediately just feel 'Oh good! That's going to be my little girl', and then I think 'Oh shit no, she's dead, she's dead' and have to remind myself.

I really do live with them in my head, and I force myself not to, too much. I've been told by therapists and friends, don't indulge in self-pity, don't indulge in pain, because you need to live your life in the present. But it's very hard. It's a daily battle. The time that you find me at now, it's raw. It's like I'm in a butcher's shop, and I'm surrounded by raw meat, and if I could just get out into the garden where the flowers are, and not deal with the meat of pain and misery, or deal with it a bit each day, but not all day every day.

Grief can also be cumulative, tapping into earlier losses. Sue was with her partner for 19 years. She had always wanted children, but they agreed early on in their relationship that they wouldn't have children until they were financially secure. When Sue was in her late 30s, they finally reached the point where it would be feasible for her to give up work and start a family.

I was thrilled, but when I raised the subject of now we can start a family, he straight away turned round and said 'I thought you'd dropped that idea, you hadn't mentioned it for so long, and I think I'm too old now.'

After eight months of 'putting her marriage under the microscope', trying to make her relationship work, she finally decided to leave her partner. One of the things she tried, during the last few months of her relationship, was marriage guidance counselling, and then a year or so after they separated, she decided to go back into counselling:

I reached a point where I needed to go and speak to a professional last year, to deal with a whole load of issues, particularly bereavement, the loss of my dad, which, you know, 20 odd years later I still hadn't really sat down and done it. That, on top of my failed marriage and a whole load of other things.

Grief is cyclical and, while it may fade, it never really goes away. Fay put aside her dreams of having children after unsuccessful IVF and divorce ten years ago:

It's an iterative process. I don't ever go back to feeling denial, or anger, or even resistance, but I do go back to some sadness every now and then. I think that is a process that perhaps will always be there, there will be poignancy ... so I've been helping somebody choose a wedding outfit recently, for their daughter's wedding, and knowing that's something I'll never do.
   In talking even this morning, I realised that there is a huge sadness, and it won't ever go away, and perhaps it never should go away, because I need to acknowledge that's happened, and it's there, and that's part of me.

Grief can also be triggered by seemingly insignificant incidents, returning with what feels like full intensity. Lucy B talks about one such incident, where she had to leave Sunday lunch with friends when the topic of conversation would not get away from children:

Someone said about going for a walk, and I said 'Yes, I'll just go to the loo', and I just went out of the room and was crying. I went upstairs, and my husband came and found me, and I said 'I can't go back down,

I'm sorry, I'm too upset, I can't even say goodbye, I don't want to, that's it.' The straw that broke the camel's back, it's one of those little things, they were talking about sewing the name tapes into their children's school uniforms, and it was one of those things that you think I'm never going to do that. My mother probably still has my old swimming towel at home, with my name tape on it, and it's one of those little things that opened the floodgates on that particular occasion.

Getting stuck in grief

From the moment I (Rachel) heard 'No children', my world caved in. Nothing in my life up to then had prepared me for this. I felt utterly lost, at sea, in turmoil, I didn't know what to think, what to say, what to do .... As the full realisation of my situation sank in, I cried and I kept on crying. I really didn't know what else to do.

I cried for four years and, mostly, I kept my tears inside. Given I was fit, healthy, had a successful career and on paper at least a great marriage, my grief felt like a shameful secret that I needed to keep hidden from the world. Gradually, I became aware that my crying no longer brought the comfort it once had. In the early days, crying was a release when my grief got too much to bear, bringing temporary relief and some sense of peace. However, as time went on, I felt more and more weighed down by my tears. It was as if I was carrying around an enormous rucksack of sorrow, which, however much I wanted to, I just couldn't put down. I remember very clearly wanting to move on, to be happy again. At my lowest ebb, I contacted the Samaritans, but however hard I tried, I just couldn't find a way through. I was stuck in grief and I desperately wanted to stop and reclaim my life.

For some women we have talked to, the coping mechanisms we've already discussed have been enough to get them through their grief. Even where the coping mechanism is a form of denial, it can perform a useful role, providing the necessary breathing space, allowing time to heal, as the intensity of grief eventually fades to a more manageable level of sadness or regret.

Others, like me (Rachel), have found themselves stuck in grief for many years, unable to find a way through. Initially, grief can be an overwhelming, almost automatic response to the enormous, multi-faceted loss of childlessness. The fact that other people, indeed society as a whole, tend not to recognise childlessness as a loss can make it very difficult to acknowledge and accept the loss and move beyond grief.

Lucy A describes her grief on having to have a hysterectomy, and the challenge of moving beyond that grief:

I really was devastated. You can't even begin to describe the pain, and although you think you're strong, although it's been going on six years, seven years, and you say it takes five or six to get over it, as you say, you get bored with it, you get thoroughly bored with being miserable and in pain, you think 'Hang on, I'm going to have a life.' Because until you get to that, actually, it's a very destructive time, it's not good for you while you're having all those conflicting emotions still. It's destruc-tive because it's all-consuming, it's all you think of, it clouds or impacts on every judgement you make, every single judgement you make it impacts on, some more than others. I think it puts your life on hold, stops you living ... and, at the end of it, one's got to be realistic and accept the situation, eventually you've got to accept the situation and you've got to decide, you've got to plan your life without children.

Acknowledging the loss

It was important for me (Rachel) to acknowledge to myself that I had suffered a loss, even though it's difficult, when the loss is of something you've never had – no birth, no death, no anniversaries, nothing to celebrate, nothing tangible. The absence of anything tangible can increase, rather than decrease, the sense of loss, making it very difficult to even acknowledge, let alone work through.

Some women do experience their loss as a very tangible one. Clare C talks about her experience:

We went for IVF treatment and I conceived three babies, three embryos I should say. I see them as babies, as lives, and they miscarried. I was pregnant for about a fortnight, and I knew exactly when they died, because when I came downstairs and said they're dead, my husband said don't be so ridiculous, but it was just like I knew, something had been switched off.

I think there was a part of me, stiff upper lip, that didn't want to put too much emphasis on it, whereas in actual fact, it was a huge thing for me. Again, I don't think I realised it until I lost the babies and realised that I wasn't going to do it again. Again, I'm calling them babies, which puts more to them than they really were, they were embryos, so they probably weren't really alive in the full sense of the word, but to me they were, they were my potential children, they were our children. It definitely felt like a bereavement.

While Natasha's experience of IVF started successfully, with 12 embryos being created, she then suffered from ovarian hyperstimulation syndrome, and was too ill for them to be implanted. While she was in hospital recovering, a freak bacterial contamination in the laboratory destroyed all the embryos. She has really struggled to come to terms with what it is that she has lost:

I felt completely numb. I didn't cry once about it. I didn't really know how to react, because what did I lose? I lost my chance, I didn't lose babies, I didn't have a miscarriage, but then again I did lose something, they were our cells that were the potential beginnings of life. But I felt numb, through the whole thing. I'm still, I don't really know ... it's not like, I can't put it in any place, it's not a bereavement, it's not a ... what is it? I don't know what it is, I can't even tell you what it is; it's like a weird thing. My husband, I think, feels the same. It's like, you tell the story to people and they're like 'Oh, what a horrible story', but what is it? No one died. We didn't have even a miscarriage, it wasn't ... you know, what is it? That's the kind of dilemma.

I can talk about it, but I can't really put it anywhere in my head. I don't really know what to do with it, if that makes sense. It just becomes this issue that is unresolved, and I'm very, very uncomfortable with things not being resolved. For me, just to have that hanging there is awful.

Helen's husband has two children from a previous marriage and had a vasectomy before they met. Although they have jointly decided that he will not have the vasectomy reversed, Helen is still able to acknowledge her loss:

It's a sense of loss, but it's a loss of something you never had. I do think it's a little bit of a bereavement of that loss. What would they have looked like? What would they have been like? Would they have looked like me, or would they have looked like my husband? Whose personality would they have had? Would they have had his incredible patience? That bit intrigues me, and I feel sad about that, the loss of that potential person in the world and what they would have been like.

Although women can experience the losses of childlessness in very different ways, acknowledging these losses can be a very important stage in the process of moving through grief.

Mourning the loss

As well as acknowledging the loss, it can also be important to mourn the loss, and the difficulty here lies in the fact that it is a lost future, rather than a lost past. It's a case of mourning the never born.

Debbie's husband already had grown-up children from a previous marriage and was clear from the start of their relationship that he didn't want any more children:

For me, the most important thing to realise was that although you can't ever talk about it with anyone, you have to do that mourning something you haven't had. Which I think is difficult, because you haven't got an object to place the affection on. My sister's son recently died, and she went and smelled his clothes. Well, I've got nothing to smell, I can't ask for anyone's sympathy, really. I haven't lost anything, I just never had it. I think nobody knows how to help you do something that you never had. It's a very lonely journey.

For me (Rachel), the breakthrough came totally unexpectedly during a counselling session when, out of nowhere, I heard myself saying that a part of me viewed Douglas as a mass murderer, who'd killed our children. I found my totally unpremeditated accusation startling, even frightening. Did I really think that? Well, he had prevented their birth; that was certainly true. It was thinking around this accusation that led me to realise that I needed to mourn the children I would never have if I was to break free of my grief. It was a seminal moment that helped me move on from the ultimate futility of endless tears to taking my first steps forward. For the first time in four years I felt in control, no longer just a helpless sobbing mass, but a woman with a clear path ahead of her. I knew it wouldn't be easy, but I felt I had been given the wherewithal to get my life and my marriage back on track.

Seeing my childlessness in terms of a bereavement felt right and strangely comforting. It reflected the magnitude of my loss, and made sense of the very strong emotions that had imprisoned me for so long. It also forced me to face my situation; I was and always would be childless. But most importantly, bereavement is a well-trodden path, providing me with a variety of possible routes out of grief.

I read lots of books on the subject. After feeling so alone for so long, it was very reassuring to find the emotions that had threatened my sanity described as normal reactions, and to realise I had already moved some way down the mourning road, with guidance on the way ahead.

I came to realise that my goal shouldn't be to 'get over' my childlessness, impossible in any case, but slowly to learn to live with it, to accept my fate and begin to think about life beyond being a non-mother. I also learnt there was no set period for mourning and no right way of dealing with all the different emotions I felt. It was also reassuring to learn that it was normal, not a sign of failure, for grief you thought you'd dealt with to reappear totally unexpectedly and very powerfully, demanding to be worked through all over again.

Childlessness as bereavement

While seeing childlessness as bereavement will not feel appropriate or helpful for every childless woman, for me (Rachel) it offered a very meaningful, useful way of being able to move through my grief and, in time, move on in life. It was very healing for me to acknowledge my anger and rage, as well as my sorrow. My approach to grieving was essentially a private one – reading books on bereavement, and reflecting on my own loss in that context. However, although I was not aware of it at the time, there are now public approaches to such grieving available, both religious and secular, which some people may find helpful.

Mourning rituals

One such ceremony is the Buddhist ritual of *Mizuko kuyo*. Literally translated, *Mizuko* means 'water baby' and is a description of the unborn, beings that float in a watery world, awaiting birth. *Mizuko kuyo* refers to a memorial service for infants who have died either before birth or within the first few years of life when their hold on life within the human realm is considered tenuous. Traditionally, grieving women sew bright red bibs, which are presented as a symbolic offering to a statue of Jizo, a monk with a baby face who protects travellers, including those who are journeying into and out of life. Although the majority of these ceremonies take place in Japan, we have read of them being organised in the US, and they may well be organised in other parts of the world.

Meredith Wheeler, a transpersonal psychotherapist, organises workshops and non-denominational memorial services in the UK for those trying to come to terms with fertility losses (see Appendix 1 for details). Her emphasis is on breaking the silence – telling our stories, naming and honouring our losses in a safe compassionate atmosphere. In an article for the *Journal of Fertility Counselling*, she describes the first memorial service in detail, including a prayer 'whose central point was the hope that our fertility experiences, however sad, would open our hearts in compassion, rather than close them in bitterness'.

Some women have also organised their own personal memorial rituals, with the assistance of a sympathetic priest, rabbi or vicar.

Even if it doesn't feel helpful to think of your loss in terms of bereavement, there may be other important rituals in letting go of grief, or reminders to grief. Penny B has one daughter and desperately wanted to have more. She spent five years trying, including IVF, and continued to grieve for a further five years. For Penny and her husband, one important step on the road to recovery was deciding to give their daughter's cot and baby clothes to a charity that supports children affected by radiation in Chernobyl:

I said 'Right, I'm going to ring them up, and they can take all the cot and everything else like that.' I remember, it was an old ambulance that they used to cart it around, and a lovely couple arrived to collect it. I remember Ken sort of throwing everything in the back of the thing, and I just wanted to say 'Ken, that's my dreams, just treat them gently, those are my dreams that are going.' I remember watching it go, and just sobbing.

Strangely, my husband was driving down the motorway. The ambulance passed him, with the Chernobyl thing, and it was the ambulance with our cot inside. He said he had to pull over, he couldn't drive, his eyes were just full of tears and he just watched this ambulance drive by, thinking, that's it, they go away.

Other aids to mourning

If the idea of a public ritual doesn't appeal to you, it can still be very helpful to talk about your loss. A large number of the women we talked to commented spontaneously that they found the process of sharing their stories with us very useful, being able to talk about their experience in a way that they had never done before.

Professional counselling

Many of the women we talked to have found professional counselling enormously beneficial. Jennie Hunt, Senior Infertility Counsellor at the IVF Unit of Hammersmith Hospital, talks here about how it can help:

One of the helpful aspects of counselling is that counsellors don't leap in with reassurance. There is something about being involved in expressing whatever your feelings are, whether they're anxiety, fear, despair, anger, whatever it is, and for once not having someone who tries to dampen those emotions, but simply acknowledges them for what they are. This tends to bring some level of relief.

There's also something about being able to hear oneself; very often this helps us to tease out exactly what we are feeling, and then it becomes a bit more manageable. Because sometimes a bad feeling gets attached to everything, everything is awful, and a counsellor can help you to focus and to be able to recognise the things that might not be so awful, so that you get perspective. Then you feel a little bit more in control, because there *are* some good things in life, not everything's awful and it's not quite so overwhelming.

The minute people can see what the problems are, I find they are so resourceful about mobilising ways of helping themselves. With a counsellor to support them, to stay with them, maybe to help them keep the focus, and sometimes to raise possibilities by asking questions, people will very often say 'No, I hadn't actually thought of that, how crazy, that's so obvious.' They've been stuck, and by just offering the right sort of query, people usually find their own solutions.

Close friends suggested counselling when they saw how distressed I (Rachel) was at being childless, but for years I rejected the idea. I saw myself as strong, competent and highly efficient, I felt I could and I would crack this one myself, I didn't need to pay someone to listen to me! I saw counselling as being for the weak, neurotic, dysfunctional, self-obsessed – life's failures. The very thought of seeing a counsellor filled me with dread and shame.

It was only when my GP recommended I talk to someone that I felt willing to accept it might help. By then, I'd lived with my childlessness for over four years, and seemed no nearer to finding any peace or resolution.

I found talking to the counsellor incredibly useful. The sessions really helped me to start to turn my life around. I'm so thankful I had the courage to put aside my prejudices, and give it a go.

As Lucy B's experience shows, counselling can provide a safe space for saying things that you can't say to a partner, friend or family member:

I think I realised that I desperately needed somebody. I did it on my own. I knew that my husband wouldn't like the idea, because he's a very private person, and wouldn't like to think of my problems, which are our problems, which are therefore his problems, being discussed with a stranger. He didn't want to come, I didn't feel I needed him to come, and the counsellor never suggested it, so it was very much my time. It was very much my space that I could say these things which I couldn't say to him or to my mother or to my sister, because they were so black and hurtful that it was good to get them out to a complete stranger. It was months; if not a year, it was quite a long time.

Tracey has known since before her 16th birthday that she wouldn't be able to have children naturally. Her pain has intensified since she met her husband five years ago, and married him just over a year ago, and has been made even worse by her husband's daughter and her own half-sister both having babies recently. She cries as she tells her story:

On New Year's Day I took an overdose. I didn't want to die, it was just because I was hurting so much. I think I just wanted to show my husband, to show everyone just how much the pain was causing me, that I couldn't do this. Yet I wanted it so much and nobody realised how I was feeling – that was really hard.

Now I've been to counselling and it's all behind me. I feel a lot stronger person now. She explained you're not a bad person to be jealous, society sees it as such a bad word they don't like to talk about it. But she explained it's just another emotion, like happiness or sadness. So I began to come to terms with not feeling bad about myself for feeling jealous, and that helped a lot. To realise I was allowed to feel jealous, it was OK, that helped a lot.

For Rebecca A, who was bullied into having an abortion by her married lover, finding a good counsellor was literally a lifeline:

I was suicidal for about a year. All I could think about was dying. If I wasn't such a coward, I would not be alive now. If I wasn't such a coward, and if I hadn't met such a good counsellor who helped me find green shoots. But I was in a bad way, didn't cope with anything in life, including my work, which went to pieces. I tried to pretend there was nothing the matter, which didn't help.

I never thought I'd be able to admit it, I suppose good things have come out of it, only because I had the counselling, I don't think the good things would have come about if I hadn't had such a magnificent counsellor. And I only wish that I'd realised 15 years ago that actually you could see a counsellor without being in a crisis, that actually it's a very healthy thing to do, to talk to somebody about you and your image of yourself and what you would like to be, the person you would like to be. I wish I'd known that, because I don't think I would have been in this long relationship [with a married man] if I'd had counselling, proper counselling, and I might have children now.

Support groups
Support groups can be very helpful in putting you in touch, either face to face or electronically, with other women in a similar situation, particularly if you're feeling isolated with nobody to talk to. Lucy B, who talked about counselling providing a safe space, describes the Daisy Network as one of her lifelines:

To go into a room and see these other women who looked perfectly normal, who I'd never have dreamed were menopausal, and to hear their stories, was good. Otherwise, it's the 'Why me? This is the worst thing that could ever happen to anybody, nobody's got a worse story than mine.' But listening to these other women and hearing their different stories made me realise that, 'OK, mine's pretty bad but so are theirs, and it's not just me.' They look normal, and they're managing.

Tracey, who talked earlier about taking an overdose as a cry for help, is hoping to have a baby through surrogacy, and has found the support of the surrogacy organisation invaluable:

For us, surrogacy is the only chance we've got and for a lady to do that for us is amazing. I just want to be a mum so much, it'd make my life complete. It's changed my view of myself, I don't feel so down on myself any more. I don't feel such an inadequate person any more. I used to be so down on myself, thinking I was worthless. Now I know there are lots of reasons why you can't have children and I'm not the only person in the world. It's been counselling in itself just to join Surrogacy UK and meet other people. It's made me feel I'm not alone; other women have been through what I've gone through. I feel stronger, more able to cope with it all.

Anne B regrets not having found a support group that would have allowed her to talk through her pain as much as she needed to, with people in a similar situation, without worrying about boring her friends and family:

People around you, however sorry they feel for the situation, because it's not them, they're not going to feel like you do about things. I think it is such a good thing to be able to talk to people who are in the same position as you, who you feel you share a common goal with. Therefore it doesn't matter how long and often you talk about it, and you can get it all out, you don't have to bottle it all up. If I could go back, I would. I did know I should do it then, but you see I'm a roughty-toughty policewoman, who doesn't do things like that. I bottled it up because I had to, because I couldn't bore people to tears about it. I'd recommend anyone to at least try going to a self-help group, with people who are in a similar position to you, who have lost babies, or can't have babies. There are two issues with me: it's not just that I haven't got any, it's that I lost one. It is two different issues.

Every time you go down the supermarket, you see people with children, and you think 'Oh, I'd love a child, I'd love a baby.' Everyone who wants children, and hasn't got them must think that. Who can you talk about that to? How can you say 'I went down the supermarket today and I saw this baby ...' You can't, who can you talk to about it? We don't want to bore people to death, and people wouldn't really understand.

Friends or family

Many of us don't find it easy to talk about our childlessness with friends or family and, when we do, the response is not always helpful. However, those women who have been able to find a sympathetic and supportive ear have generally found it very helpful.

Sam is a Muslim, originally from Pakistan:

I can talk about this [with my female friends]. It helps me. When I talk to anyone about any worries, and also about the babies as well, and when I cry, after this I feel better. Otherwise I feel all the burden, it's like I'm holding everything with me, and when I talk to someone I feel totally relaxed, but only for maybe one day or a few days, after this I've got all this again and I need to just get it out.

For Helen, having a sister-in-law who can't have children helps her to feel less isolated, particularly at social gatherings:

Interestingly, one of my brothers is married to someone who had cancer and can't have children. That's quite nice, having a sister-in-law that can't have children, because we often use each other for moral support, particularly if we're at events with all of our mutual girlfriends and the conversation is all about children. She and I will go into a corner and huddle, talk about other things and such like.

For Linda, who had one daughter and was unable to have any more children, finding other people in her family with similar experiences helped her to feel less alone:

It helped me, finding out that I had two cousins to whom I'm very close, and they both had exactly the same thing, had one child and then never got pregnant again. And that my sister had trouble, she did conceive a second time, but seven or eight years later, so her kids are eight years apart. It made me at least feel as though it wasn't so ... odd, different.

And for Marilyn, talking to an old friend who doesn't have children has given her a positive role model, helping her to recognise that there is the possibility of happiness, even if she ultimately remains childless:

I talk a lot to an old school friend who was a headmistress and has then done a counselling course. I talk to her a lot; she's been through everything in my life. She's not married, she didn't want children, she's a mother to the world, and when she gets to her own house she wants to shut the doors and shut us all out and get on with it. She helps a lot, because that's a different life, a different successful life, to the ones that have got children. She's perfectly happy with what she's done, she's doing what she wants to do, and she's extremely successful, so that's good.

Some of the women we spoke to have found that writing about their feelings of loss, whether it be in the form of a journal, or in the form of a letter to the child or children they will never have, can play an important part in acknowledging and accepting their pain and their loss.

As Virginia Ironside says in her excellent book on bereavement, *You'll Get Over it*:

> *Talking or writing about the death is one way of trying to regain control (...) Telling people is not always just born out of a desire to talk things out, or a desire for sympathy, or as a way of getting the truth to sink slowly in. It's a way of clawing back the power into your life. You have no power over the death, but you do have power over the story.*

Forgiveness

Being able to forgive – whether yourself, your partner, a family member, friends, a doctor – takes practice. It's a decision, not a feeling. For me (Rachel), it's taken many years of working at it, and I'm not totally there yet. Douglas was the person I most needed to forgive for not wanting children – the survival of our marriage depended on it.

I've had to dig deep inside myself to understand and support Douglas, because the last thing I wanted was to stay married to him and be bitter and twisted. So I had to somehow come to terms with his decision and to love him for what he is. If not wanting children was part of him, I had to learn to love that part of him, too, which was very difficult. But I can honestly say now that I look on that aspect of him as just a part of him, like the fact he wears glasses. It's neither good nor bad, it's just him.

Of course, even when you love someone there's going to be elements of them that you really adore, elements that drive you nutty, and elements that you really could just do without – it's all part of the package. As I see it, you have to learn to love every bit of them and I've had to learn to accept the bit that really wounded me.

I needed to forgive myself, too, for marrying someone who it turned out didn't want children. I've also had to forgive a host of family, friends and acquaintances who, over the years, have said things that, totally unbeknown to them, hurt and which I'd stored away, increasing the hurt. If I was to move on, I realised I had to let go of it all.

Moving beyond grief

Acknowledging that there has been a loss, real and painful, even if intangible, and reconciling yourself to the reality of that loss are important steps in being able to let go, and move beyond grief. For me (Rachel) it was important to realise that my goal was not to 'get 'over' my childlessness, but gradually to learn to live with it.

It's now five years since Eve had two unsuccessful cycles of IVF:

I think it's just time, really. It's that old saying, time heals everything and it does. I think just common sense, just by realising, well, it's not going to change. Just time, I suppose.

I didn't talk to my friends that much about it: one girlfriend in particular, and one male friend who works for the Samaritans. That was it, really. Most of the time I would just sort of sit and moan and cry, things like that. It didn't last that long, actually, I think I got my head round it probably quite quickly. I know people think I got my head round it a lot quicker than I actually did, I was very good at just keeping it under wraps, but then somebody would say one thing and that would set me off.

That makes it sound like an illness ... which it sort of is, really, it kind of is an illness. It's an illness which has a cure, if you want it. The illness was just like the illness in your head and in your heart, and the cure, I don't know what the cure was really ... time. A cure that can only come from yourself, nobody else can make you get better. You can go and have counselling until you're blue in the face, but you're the one that's got to get your head around it. I suppose I did it myself, really.

My aim in life is not to get over it, it's to deal with it the best way that I can. Because I don't think it's something that should be got over. It's quite an important part of my life. I feel it's a part of me, and it's probably helped in making me what I am now. I don't think I'll ever get over it, I'll get used to it. I'm not 100 per cent there yet, but I am getting used to it. It will always be there, and I will never forget it.

Although Heather doesn't belong to any particular religious group, she does come from a religious background, which has helped her to view her childlessness with a fatalistic perspective:

If that's the way it is for me, that's the way it is. It's the same for lots of other things that happen to you in life and you learn to live with it, rather than anything else. I think (my childlessness) is probably now like other things. At a different level, I'm as blind as a bat, and you learn how to cope with that, what aids to have, like contact lenses, to make sure that you can see when you need to be able to see. In a way, it's finding whatever the mechanisms are to help you cope at the time you have to cope. The sight is a physical thing, the childlessness is physical, but much more an emotional thing.

For Lesley, it's about living in the present:

I think you need to learn to live in the present and live in acceptance, and that's kind of a broader thing than just childlessness, that's something to do with life. I don't know if you've read *The Power of Now*, there's a lot of stuff being written like that. It is absolutely futile to live in the past and regret the past, it doesn't mean that we don't all do it, because we do, but I think all you can really do with it is look at it and try to learn from it. The issue is not to sit in it ... yes, you have to go through anger, grief, all the rest of it, but it is to say, 'This is the situation as it is today; what am I now going to do with it?' Not wallow in regrets, because it gets you and nobody else anywhere. I increasingly try to live my life that way, and that of course helps with it hugely.

It's over ten years since Fay's unsuccessful attempt at IVF, and as she goes through the menopause she reflects again on her childlessness:

There's almost a state of grace, I want to say, which is a bit old fashioned, and in some ways friends would laugh if they heard me say that. I have every intention of being a complete barmy old woman, but there is this state of grace ... it's about, and when I say coming to maturity I don't mean emotional maturity, necessarily, my body's maturing and is saying to me this is what's happening now, and again you have no control. You have two options, don't you, you live through it or you don't live through it. So the option is you live through it.

It's about saying I am this woman, and there are other women who've had different experiences, and OK I didn't have that experience but I now know I'm no less a woman for it. I'm a different woman...

But moving beyond grief, and starting to think in terms of what life still has to offer, as opposed to what you have been denied, is not an easy task. As Liz Scott, Fertility Counsellor at the Assisted Conception Unit of the Lister Hospital, says:

I think it's a very isolating and very individual experience that so many people carry, which increases the difficulty and the pain around it. I think this issue of moving on with childlessness is one that hasn't been dealt with very well, and is such a difficult area. It's like that black hole, that yawning void that opens up before patients that's too dreadful to think about. It's just the terror for a lot of people that we work with, they cannot visualise it, life without children, it's just unimaginable, they can't go there. I'm hoping that what your book will provide is an acknowledgement of that journey, and that people manage it, and that people come out the other side and that people don't disintegrate.

I really encourage women to look at this, that this looks so finite, at the end, this is where the terror is, but in fact there's a whole new life but it's about getting through the losses first, and the pain, and then being able to invest that energy and say 'Yes, there is another world out there and another life.' If they can begin to recognise that there is a life out there, earlier on, that's what I'm encouraging people to do.

But, ultimately, moving on is a choice. As John Welshons says, in his book *Awakening from Grief*:

> More than anything, we need to remember that when our hearts are broken, they are also wide open. Our task is to fill the openness with love, awareness and compassion, not to fill it with bitterness and self pity. Ultimately, it's our choice. And ultimately, the recognition must be that there is no payoff in spending our lives feeling victimized.

CHAPTER 10

Alternative nurturing

We have already seen that for many of us the need or desire to nurture is strong. As Lucy A says:

It comes back to this need that a woman has. You are instilled with this need to nurture, to love, to care, to teach – we put it all under one banner of mothering.

If we can't have children of our own, there are a number of ways in which this desire may be fulfilled – through alternative forms of parenting, through relationships with other people's children or through other forms of loving and caring.

Alternative parenting

For many women, exploring the alternatives for parenting is a natural next step after discovering that they cannot have children of their own. The main alternatives are adoption, either within the UK or from overseas, and surrogacy. Just like fertility treatments, these are not options for the faint-hearted. There are no guarantees and the probability of actually 'taking delivery' of a baby is relatively low. Both adoption and surrogacy involve complex processes that can be incredibly stressful, onerous and lengthy, testing your desire for a child to the limits. For many couples, the process inevitably becomes the main focus in life, for years rather than months, with other aspects of life having to be put on hold.

Elizabeth is one of the lucky ones, with her son born last year as a result of surrogacy. Here, she reflects on the nature of the process:

It places a tremendous strain on your relationship. To some extent, we've felt in limbo the last couple of years, and unable to plan for anything because of what's been going on. The whole process was actually really quite quick for us, it was two and a half years. That was partly because, after meeting our surrogate, seven months after we met her, she was pregnant, which is incredible, really. It absolutely couldn't have been quicker, because you have to go through certain tests, and counselling, and then you have to start the IVF treatment ... I'm pretty sure you couldn't hope to do it much more quickly than that. You do read about couples that have spent six years, literally – they've met surrogates, the relationship's broken down, they try to find some-body else, they go through various rounds of treatment ...

In this chapter, it's not our intention to explore the detailed practical, ethical, legal, financial and, in the case of surrogacy, medical processes involved. Instead, what we aim to do is to provide an insight into some of the emotional challenges of the processes so that if you are considering adoption or surrogacy you will be better informed and can make the decision that is right for you, or if you have already been through the experience, you can perhaps feel less isolated, reading of other women's experiences.

Exploring the possibilities

For many women who want a child, it can feel useful if not essential to explore all the possible alternative options before feeling able to face the possibility of childlessness. For Elizabeth, who talked above about feeling in limbo, this was definitely the case:

It [surrogacy] was something that I felt I wanted to explore in more detail. I'm very much somebody who always wants to have the approach to life that's 'No regrets', and so I suppose I felt at that stage that if I explored all of the options open to me to have children and actually nothing came of it, then that was fine, and I could live with what was destined for me, but I felt that I wouldn't be able to rest until I'd done that.

Partners' views

Many of the women we spoke to had been able to make the journey from wanting their own biological child, to wanting a child they can love, nurture and raise, even if it is not biologically theirs. Judy's view is quite typical:

It's been a very interesting journey. You start in one place, then you end up somewhere quite different. In the beginning, your priority about having a child is that it has to be your own child, with your own genes, and all the rest of it. Then, when you have infertility treatment, you think this is not actually going to be a natural child, the process is so unnatural. Then you reject a lot of things like donor eggs, because you think that wouldn't even be our child. Then going down the adoption route seems very alien. Then as you really think about it, you learn to understand that it's really about a child, and that is more important than whether the child is from your gene pool or not.

However, partners may not necessarily feel the same way.

For some men, like Lucy B's husband, it may simply be a gut feeling, which in Lucy's case reinforced her own ambivalence about adoption:

My husband didn't want to adopt, he had a gut feeling about it. I think I could have come round to the idea, but he had a gut feeling about it, and I thought if you have a feeling like that about it, then that is not something to be talked out of, just to try and please me. I thought it would be wrong of me to do that, and to put him under pressure to do that.

For others, like Anne A's husband, it was a lack of conviction:

We did talk about children, because he knew I would have very much loved to have children. We did speak about adoption, and he said 'Well look, I know how much you want children, and if that's what you want, I'll go with it.' But I felt he wasn't as enthusiastic as I was, so in the end I thought 'Well I don't want to spoil my marriage.' Even though I wanted children so much, I didn't want to press adoption if he didn't feel 100 per cent behind me. So we decided that was it.

For some men, like Sally's husband, Jock, who supported his wife through four unsuccessful cycles of IVF, it's the potential hassle, trouble and heartache of adoption and surrogacy, and the fact that these routes can feel very alien, that is particularly off-putting:

While all that [the IVF] was going on, I was having to work out in my mind, if it came to the point where we'd failed, I wouldn't be into surrogacy, because Sally had talked about surrogacy as well, I was having none of that. I just felt trouble after trouble, trouble x 10, heartache x 15, going down the surrogacy route. Heartache, potentially, x 5 going down the adoption route. I thought, right, we'll put 110 per cent into it [the IVF], we're fortunate enough to have the money, the backing of the doctor, young enough to persevere through the whole thing. If it doesn't work, OK, I'm a very practical guy, we'll have a super life and spend all our dosh on good food, holidays and so on. The world won't come to an end if we don't have a child.

I think men can look at the hassle factor more than the joy factor. Men take a more practical view of life, sometimes, and say 'Look this is going to be a problem, a headache. The headache factor here will be high, so let's not even go near it.' If inevitably you're going to have a headache, why have a headache if you can avoid it?

A fellow, not having his wife as the baby provider, that's just so bloody alien, it's way out there on the shelf somewhere, it's like IVF used to be, funny. Funny, funny, funny. It's unnatural, it's off the wall, it's very lateral; it's a solution but it's so lateral that you can't actually take yourself through it and think about it.

Linda has one daughter and would have loved more. She believes that her husband, whose sperm is low in motility, was reluctant to adopt because somehow it would have felt like an admission of failure:

I really wanted to adopt, but he didn't want to. I didn't realise until much later but I think because it would be saying to the world that he was a failure. I felt as though I had to protect him, I never talked about it, I never mentioned it, I never said a word to anybody. I just said I didn't want any more children, that we had decided that one was enough with our lifestyle.

I felt terrible, I felt as though I was lying all the time. I was lying to myself, I was lying to everybody else, really just to protect him. But in protecting him, I suppose I was protecting myself. I probably didn't really want people to know that my husband was defective. So it was as important for me to protect his image as it was for him to be protected.

For some men, such as Sam's husband, who is from Pakistan, a reluctance to adopt is about not trusting themselves to love a child that isn't biologically theirs:

My husband, he's not ready to adopt a son or daughter. He says 'I don't mind if a child comes into my house and we could do whatever we could do for him, but I have no trust in myself maybe later on. Now we need a baby, we are desperate to have a baby, we get the baby, we play with him, after a while we maybe get fed up and I can't be as a father like I can be a father to my real child. This is not fair on the child, and I don't want to do this with any child. That's why I can't trust myself. I've got the feeling at the moment, but maybe later on I will change, that is not fair to the child.'

Interestingly, this is a view that some women share. Natasha has one son, aged 6, and despite trying for a baby for the last three years, including undergoing IVF treatment, she has not been able to have another child:

People have said to us, 'Why don't you adopt a second child?', but I think that if you have one natural child it's very hard. For me, I don't think I could trust myself to have had the same unconditional love and devotion for an adopted second child, which was sitting alongside a natural child. I think that would have been very, very difficult for me. Because I'm an honest person to myself, I think that I would always fear that at some point in my life I would judge that child to not be the same or equal. Which would have been different if I'd had, say, two adopted children.

Going through the process

For both surrogacy and adoption, the processes can take many years, and be very stressful, with ultimately no guarantee of success.

For Sally, it was the prospect of another lengthy process, which might fail, after years of unsuccessful fertility treatments that put her off seriously pursuing the adoption route:

I know people who've adopted and it's worked out great. I think maybe we should have had a bit more courage and really pushed for it, but the other thing that I couldn't bear at the time was failure and rejection. Having failed and failed and failed at this (IVF), if you put yourself forward as adoptive parents, you get assessed, and you get tested, and I just didn't want to go through a whole set of tests and then they turn round and say 'No, you're not right', it just seemed too hard. By this time we were in our late 30s: if I had been 28 not 38 then I think we would have looked at adoption, we would have had more time. The very idea of being five years on a waiting list, and being tested and assessed without much hope of a positive outcome...

Lucy A and her husband spent several years going through the process for adoption. For Lucy, the prospect of ongoing contact with the adopted child's birth family was one of the major factors that made her decide not to proceed:

We didn't really like the idea, that the adoption system these days is that the child has to know very early on that they're adopted. The grandparents, the family, you have to send them a letter once or twice a year telling them about the child, a photograph, you must allow them to see them occasionally if they want, you keep in touch. In the end you're thinking 'Hang on, I'm not actually going to be a parent here, I'm just an unpaid nanny.' You know; if they're that keen to keep in touch, why are they not looking after the child themselves? But that's the way the system is.

This constant having to keep in touch, we couldn't actually break free and be our own family, and have a proper, intimate family life, there were always going to be people looking over your shoulder, who you're answerable to. I've met people who have adopted, and I've seen what they have to go through, and I just think 'No, if I'm going to do this, it's got to be mine, and if I can't have mine, then you get on with your life, I can't do it.'

Judy and her husband are still going through the process to adopt a child:

I said to my husband a few months back 'What do you think about this, we've got to make decisions about all of this, we've got to decide where we're going to adopt from, you're not being any help.' It was lovely, he said 'Judy, I don't know how to put this but if you put a little baby in front of me now, or a child, and said "Will you adopt that child?", I would pick it up and adopt it without hesitation. But this process is so overwhelming that it just destroys all of my energy.' So that was good, that made me feel a lot better. I feel exactly the same way, if the truth be known.

Jane B adopted her two sons as babies almost 20 years ago, but she still remembers the process vividly:

The process is, I think, one of the most appalling processes there is. You go once a week, and you're chatting amongst these people that you don't really know, and you're being judged for the whole time as to whether or not you are able to bring up a family. That was a horrid feeling. You'd go each week, and they'd talk to you and you'd have to talk back, and they'd have people in who would say all the pros about having adoption and then all the things that could go horribly wrong and whether or not you could have a black baby or a white baby, whether you wanted an older child.

Then, after all these weeks and weeks and weeks of going to have these talks, you then get an assessor who then comes to your home and you go through more and more and more talks about your attitudes and everything. Unbelievable. Hours, she'd come for two hours on a Monday night and just sit and interview us. Just outrageous really, the process.

Not everyone finds the process such a negative experience. Alice and her husband, who adopted two sons who are now in their teens, actually found the process very helpful:

I think it's a very useful process, because it raises issues which perhaps you haven't thought through, and in the course of thinking those through, I think we came closer and found ourselves more and more in accord on the whole than we had been.

And for Caroline and her husband, who have adopted their two children from overseas, it was a very positive experience after years of failed fertility treatments:

I was quite excited about [going down the adoption route]. I sort of felt that at last there was something that we could do, that we were more in control. With things like IVF, you're not really in control of your body, it's either going to work or it's not going to work, there's not that much extra you can do. Whereas I felt with the adoption thing, we could control it more. If we put the effort in, we would get our children.

I now say to people who are going through IVF, just forget it; just go for adoption. I know that IVF does work, but actually, in an awful lot of cases it doesn't work, and you could adopt a child who ... you know, I can't really see the difference between adoption and birth.

Elizabeth talked earlier about feeling in limbo during the surrogacy process. Here, she goes on to talk in more detail about how daunting she and her husband found the process initially, until they were able to break it down into more manageable chunks:

We started seriously looking at what options were open to us. At first, we thought very briefly about surrogacy. It was so difficult to find information about it, and also there are such hugely negative attitudes towards surrogacy in the UK, it's very much seen as an underground, slightly shady procedure. We got in touch with COTS, who are a surrogacy organisation, and they sent us some forms with a million tests that we needed to have, and crime checks and all the rest of it, and I have to be honest and say we looked at it and felt hugely daunted ... So you have crime tests on you, HIV tests, all sorts of things before you even join the organisation.

Eventually, about a year after I got the first forms through, we actually completed them and sent them back. While we were on the COTS waiting list, because they had a huge lack of surrogates, and there just didn't seem to be anything happening, we started having our first interviews for adoption and the social worker said, 'You're so young to adopt, why not consider surrogacy?' I think I was really overwhelmed by it, I couldn't find any information about it, you don't exactly meet people who've done surrogacy. I honestly think that I just felt so overwhelmed by the whole issue that I didn't seriously consider it, and it was only once we started moving slowly along the process that actually you realise it is much easier than you think. It's like anything; if you break it into bite-sized chunks it all becomes much more manageable.

Adoption, the reality

As we have seen above, the process for assessment as potential adoptive parents can be very lengthy. However, when the actual adoption happens, it can happen very quickly indeed.

Alice, who talked earlier about finding the assessment process very helpful, was in a state of shock when her older son arrived:

It all happened drastically quickly. We were phoned on Monday night to say that we were on a shortlist of three couples, and the adoption panel was meeting on the Tuesday morning. We were phoned on Tuesday to say that the adoption panel had chosen us. I was at my desk at work at 8:30 on Wednesday morning, writing out a list of the things I had to do that day; that was my last day in the office. On Thursday morning I sat with a baby book making a shopping list, and Thursday afternoon we went to buy the baby goods. Then Friday morning, I went to a bottle feeding class at the local clinic, Friday afternoon we drove down to [the birth mother's home], Saturday we met our son and Sunday we brought him home. Monday was a public holiday, but on Tuesday morning my husband left for the office and I was alone with a 6-week-old baby.

It was a complete shock, really, whereas I think if you had nine months, you've got more time to prepare.

Not having nine months to prepare was not the only disadvantage that Alice found of not having been pregnant:

Our friends were scattered all over London, so I didn't have much of a local network. I think that makes a huge difference, really, as compared to a more normal initiation into motherhood, because you would be part of a National Childbirth Trust group, or something like that, which is a local group. I still come across parents of people in my son's year at school, now that he's already 16, and we get talking about local people and she'll say 'Oh yes, I was in the same NCT group.' So I didn't have that network of local mums.

Alice also found that it took longer to bond with her son than she had expected:

My first feeling, if I think about it, was actually tremendous pride in my baby. He was a very sweet baby, seemed to be quite bright, and alert, and I think it came from the very start. It was later that the other big feeling, which is the protective feeling, came round. Initially the protective thing was more of a chore and a duty; I think that's probably how it felt to me. One did it out of duty and only as the bonding process went along did it become protection out of love. I guess the bonding process did take longer because this was adoption, and probably because of having to adjust my own life so sharply.

She also attributes the continuing bad relations between her two sons to the abrupt nature of the adoption process:

I have two sons that don't get on, and I had expected the siblings to get on. I suspect that at the beginning of this, this is partly to do with the abruptness of adoption in that my younger son suddenly arrived in the house at 20 months, running and kicking and up to all sorts of dastardly things, so that I couldn't take my eyes off him for more than two seconds.

My older son, who was then 5, found it very difficult to cope with this. If I'd had a baby myself, that baby would have arrived, would have spent a lot of time sleeping, wouldn't have been running all around the place to start off with, and I think that baby's arrival would have been much easier for the older sibling. I often suspect that the continuing bad relations between my boys goes back to that.

Another issue mentioned by a number of the women we spoke to who had adopted children was that family, friends and even acquaintances feel free to share their views on all aspects of adoption, regardless of how hurtful this can be. Caroline's experience is typical:

It's interesting isn't it, friends kept saying 'Oh, but when you adopt, you'll probably get pregnant naturally', and that used to make me really cross. After we had our daughter, people would say that, and I would say 'But adoption is not a form of fertility treatment, ooh let's adopt one, so I can give birth to one.' [It annoyed me] because it was almost like they were trying to make out that adoption was the second-best thing, I could still have my own baby, just let's adopt one because then we can shove her into the background, be pregnant ...

Surrogacy, the reality

There are significant ethical, legal and financial issues involved with surrogacy, which we will not be addressing here. Any woman considering surrogacy would be advised to consider these issues carefully, perhaps by joining one of the surrogacy organisations (see Appendix 1). We will be focusing on the emotional issues involved, and as well as talking to women who have had children through surrogacy (and, in one case, also been a surrogate mum herself), we have also spoken to a counsellor who is experienced in this field.

The planning stage

As Jennie Hunt, Senior Infertility Counsellor at the IVF unit of Hammersmith Hospital, says, it is important to be emotionally ready to undertake surrogacy:

If someone's partner had just died, you wouldn't expect them to be able to contemplate a future where they'd meet somebody else. Not at that point in time. The pain is too great. The grief is too over-whelming. It would be offensive and shocking to suggest to somebody 'You'll meet somebody else.' We know about that. But it's very much the same for someone who's just learned that they're not going to be able to carry their own child, or be pregnant, to say 'Well don't worry, someone else will do it for you', the analogy is absolutely direct.

As Jennie goes on to say, preparation is essential:

You've got to prepare for all possible eventualities. So we have to look at what is it going to feel like if there is no pregnancy, what if there's a pregnancy and a miscarriage, what if there's a pregnancy and the surrogate wanted a termination because there was a diagnosis of abnormality, what if there was a stillbirth, what if there was a child born – despite all the testing – that had a physical disability, there are all these what ifs. There are so many things to cover. And what if the surrogate changed her mind? That has to be absolutely in the forefront. That's why couples have to be so clear about their legal position.

The other thing that's really painful about this is that we're asking them to anticipate, and to do all this work to prepare for surrogacy when we have no guarantee that they'll ever get the opportunity to experience it. Sometimes you think it's too hard to expect them to do this. And yet if you don't, people may be unprepared and less able to cope if things go wrong. Also, they may not make an emotionally informed choice unless they've thought of all the possibilities. In an ideal world you'd say we'll talk about these things if someone gets pregnant, and there is a baby to actually plan for, but they wouldn't have made an emotionally informed choice about whether to go down the road at all. The best we can do is to say we are aware that it's hard to talk about all the implications of surrogacy when one of their greatest fears is that it will never happen.

One of the major decisions at the planning stage is which type of surrogacy to have. In straight, or partial, surrogacy, the surrogate's egg is impregnated with the intended father's sperm. This is typically done at the surrogate's home, without any involvement by a fertility clinic. In host, or full, surrogacy, the egg used is that of the intended mother, who undergoes the first part of the IVF cycle to harvest her eggs. The egg is then fertilised in the lab with the intended father's sperm, and the resulting embryo(s) are implanted in the surrogate in the second part of the IVF cycle.

For Elizabeth, who talked earlier about needing to have explored all the options, and about how daunting she initially found the process, the decision was straightforward:

I was really clear that I didn't want to do straight surrogacy, which is where you use the surrogate's eggs and your husband's sperm, I was really clear that wasn't what I wanted to do.

Before Jayne decided to try surrogacy, she had already been through 12 cycles of fertility drugs, 20 cycles of fertility injections and spent a year trying to complete one cycle of IVF as cycles kept having to be abandoned:

We did think of using my eggs, because I could have had my eggs put in a surrogate. We looked into that option as well, but the doctors said IVF is such a lottery, it still might not work, and it's very expensive. The surrogate could have got pregnant with twins, and it would have been harder for her ... I just felt I couldn't have any more drugs put through me, basically, straight surrogacy was the less complicated, easier to get pregnant.

I think if a woman is going to give birth to a baby, at the end of the day, it doesn't matter whose eggs they are, she still has to go through the emotional process of surrogacy, really. We'd already looked at adoption, and this baby would be genetically related to one of us, and that was a bonus.

Tracey is in the early stages of her surrogacy journey and isn't ruling anything out:

A lot of the ladies who've tried host and it hasn't worked, they've gone for straight surrogacy. More than anything in the world, I want mine and my husband's baby, but then in the back of my mind I'm thinking, 'Could I give it a go if it wasn't part of me, if it was my husband's sperm?' But all the time, we've been 'It's got to be our baby, our baby.' So I don't know, we'll have to cross that bridge when we come to it.

Having decided what type of surrogacy to have, the next stage is to find a surrogate, and for the majority of women going down this route in the UK that will happen through one of the surrogacy organisations. Jayne, who talked above about her decision to have straight surrogacy, was very clear about the sort of surrogate she was looking for:

For me, my vision was to make a friend through surrogacy, to have a baby, but to gain a friend for life. I'm not in favour of the way it appears to be done in America, where it's very commercial. The best person to be your surrogate is your friend, or someone in the family, and for those people that don't have anybody like that, the next best is to find somebody that can become a friend, and a friend for life. Those are the best surrogacies for all involved.

Having found a surrogate, developing the relationship is very important. Jayne goes on to say:

Getting to know each other, not rushing into it, taking time, getting to know each other as friends. You would want to do your best by your best friend, you wouldn't dream of upsetting or hurting that friend in any way. I met all the family, I met my surrogate's mother, we talked about her being a surrogate, I invited my parents down before my mum died, and my mum met her. I didn't need to do that for my mum to give her the OK, it was more for my surrogate to see the type of family that we were, so she would feel happy about the type of family that this child would be brought up in, for her benefit, not for my benefit, well for all our benefits really.

Elizabeth, who opted for host surrogacy, agrees:

Every two or three weeks, we would go up and spend a weekend with our surrogate and her partner, or vice versa. It was [quite odd] to begin with, but it's almost like you hothouse friendship, and although we're very different, we come from very different backgrounds, my surrogate and I have got more in common than I would ever have thought. So it was difficult to begin with, and it felt unnatural, whereas in more recent months it didn't, and genuinely you felt that you were going to see friends.

With the law as it is in the UK, it is almost inevitable that, on some level, there will be fear that the surrogate mother will decide to keep the baby. As Elizabeth goes on to say:

It's terrible, because if you say to me, rationally, did I believe that she would keep the baby, I would have said to you 'No, 99 per cent sure', but emotionally you always have this fear. My husband and I actually talked about the worst case scenario, which would be that she kept the baby. We discussed it and said, 'Well listen, on balance, she and her partner would make really good parents,' and they would have done, that's absolutely true, and so we said 'Fine, that's a risk we're prepared to take, because we know if we bring a child into the world, even if it were to stay with them, we think that they would be good parents.' It's a really weird thing to have to think about, but I think you do, if you're looking at surrogacy you have to think about those sorts of questions.

During pregnancy

Once the surrogate mother actually gets pregnant, the pregnancy can be a challenging, as well as an exciting, time for the intended mother. Elizabeth found the lack of control very difficult:

The things that were difficult about it is you're not in control, someone else is carrying your child and, like it or not, you have to trust them and have to believe that they're doing the right thing for you because you can't be there telling them what to eat, what to do and what not to do.

She also found the level of support she felt she wanted to give to her surrogate during the pregnancy challenging:

The thing I found most difficult was the emotional support that – I wouldn't say she needed, but I felt like I owed her. The best way I can describe it is it's like having another partner, and this sounds weird, it's almost like having a partner that's slightly falling out of love with you, and you know when you feel like you've got to work really hard to try and keep a relationship going, and to make sure that person is still feeling good about you, that's what it was like, and that I found very difficult. There would be times when you would come home from work, absolutely knackered, you wouldn't want to talk to people, yet you'd always, not every day, but two or three times a week I'd be picking up the phone and finding out how she was, and giving her emotional support.

My motivation for doing that was, I suppose, so that she would know I was a good person and therefore she wouldn't keep the baby. So that's what you're doing, you're constantly trying to build and fuel that relationship so that the balance of power, which they are holding hugely, is tipped a bit more in your favour because they're thinking about what the implications would be on you if they were to do that. You're trying to create that emotional link so that it's not easy for them to turn their back and decide to just cast you aside.

For Jayne, it's about treating your surrogate how you would want to be treated yourself during the pregnancy:

You've got to be sensitive to your surrogate's feelings. She's going to be feeling quite sick at the beginning, really very tired, then at the end she's going to be feeling quite tired, so during the pregnancy, if you were pregnant, your husband would buy you flowers and chocolates and make you feel special, because you're having his child, so that's how you treat your surrogate, how you would like to be treated. It makes her feel special. If she's feeling really sick and tired and she gets a bunch of flowers, it lifts her spirits. Treat her like a queen, basically, and look after her children, maybe take her children out, get involved with her children.

After the birth

Unlike in most adoptions, with surrogacy the intended mother is involved right through the process, from before the baby is conceived to being present at the birth, and the women we spoke to had bonded almost instantly with their babies. As Jayne says:

It's as if you've given birth. As soon as the baby's born it's placed in your arms. Generally people have photographs taken with their surrogate, holding the baby, we've got photographs, and you have to make the decisions for the baby from there on in. What injections it's going to have, what sort of milk it's going to drink, some women can even actually breast feed, but it's a very complicated process. It sounded too complicated to me, and I was just happy to have a baby. I was afraid of doing it and it didn't work. I didn't feel I was missing out by not breast feeding.

For Elizabeth, whose son was 6 weeks old when we spoke to her for this book, bringing him home marked the start of feeling normal:

Since we've been home it's been so much better, because now for the first time, as much as is possible, I feel normal. People kept saying to me, 'Gosh, you must be so excited', and I'd be like 'Yeah, I am', but I always felt that I couldn't get excited until he was home and I was going through the process I suppose I'm going through now. Now, honestly, it feels like the most natural thing in the world, and people keep saying to me 'Oh you're really relaxed, really not stressed out at all', and I feel that's actually, genuinely the case, it feels really normal. I'm glad, because so much about it hasn't been.

Both Jayne and Elizabeth have ongoing relationships with their surrogates. Jayne knew right from the beginning that this was important to her:

I wanted to keep in touch with my surrogate, so that the child would grow up knowing how she was born. I just felt it was better for the child. We look at it like extended family, our surrogate's like an aunt figure, and she's very happy that way. My daughter looks on her half brothers and sisters, in the surrogate's family, as like cousins.

Jayne's feelings about her daughter growing up knowing how she was born are reinforced by Jennie Hunt, Senior Fertility Counsellor at the IVF unit of Hammersmith Hospital:

It used to be the case that the idea of sharing this information with children was pretty firmly established as something you do when a child is old enough to be interested in babies and where they come from, which is 4ish, depending on the child, and depending on the family. That thinking has really changed, and it is much more the case that people are saying don't wait at all, but talk openly with the child as a newborn baby, pre-verbal. It's not to do with the child being able to understand the words. It's two things: one, ensuring that the child never remembers being told, it's always part of their identity, which probably would be the case if you started at about 4; but the second point is to do with parents becoming so comfortable with the conversation that all trace of anxiety, all those non-verbal messages, have been wiped, because as we all know, the non-verbal messages can be more powerful than the verbal ones.

Fostering, the reality

When we started working on the book, we assumed that fostering would stand alongside adoption and surrogacy as a possible route for alternative parenting. However, in reality, despite being eligible and despite there being a national shortage of foster carers in the UK, our research suggests that very few childless women actually foster.

One who does is Maisie, who is in her mid-40s and has been fostering teenagers for five years, initially on a respite basis, then full time:

I saw an advert [for respite and part-time carers] and I felt invited, it's like 'You mean ME!' It had lesbians in there, and single people and black people, and my age ... it was just lovely. It was that advert which let me live out what I was keeping a lid on. From the jealousy, from just feeling something unlived in me, to be that person that someone would call Mum and to know what that means. To act out all the love, all the relationship stuff that had been building up. To be able to leave my own child self behind. It feels like a rite of passage. I didn't want to be thought of by myself and others as a spinster aunt for the rest of my life, and outside this exclusive parenthood club. I would have felt like an eternal child ... feeling left behind, like what do you do?

The fact that those who foster are now called foster carers, rather than foster parents, provides some insight into the challenges facing childless women who consider fostering. Meryl Sturdy, Assistant Team Manager, Fostering Recruitment, Family Placements Service, City of Westminster, explains the name change:

It's primarily to help a child's birth parents accept that their child is coming into care but that we are not intending to replace them, their role in life; and for the carer, their role is very clearly to care for someone else's children and not to try to be their parents.

It is worth bearing in mind that most children are taken into care following either abuse or neglect or both. It is crucial that the foster carer acknowledges the importance of the child's birth parents in that child's life; no matter how badly those parents may have treated the child in the past.

As Meryl Sturdy says about the relationship between foster carers and birth parents:

The best way [for foster carers] to help the child is to try to see where the parents are coming from and think positively about those parents, because that will have an impact on the child's self-esteem. We also try to help [the foster carers] understand that what they're doing is not just caring, it's professional and you may have to manage working with birth parents who are experiencing difficulties.

While it is a form of parenting, fostering is parenting in partnership, and the foster carer is only one member of the 'team'.

Meryl Sturdy talks about the emotional tightrope that foster carers have to walk:

We want [foster carers] to treat them like their own children, they get paid, but the child needs to be very much accepted into the family. So all the issues around being a mum in terms of the child belonging, feeling loved, feeling accepted, feeling someone really wants the best for them, which is what you'd want for your own children, foster carers need to provide that.

But it's a tightrope, they can't see the child as too much of a job, nor as too much their own child. There are some foster carers who would want to have complete ownership of the child, which is great in terms of giving the best care they can give them, but because of the fact that these children are 'in care', we have responsibility for the decision-making, not them, which can be difficult for some foster carers to accept.

The carer needs to work in partnership with us. You are doing the basic caring, but you've got to check everything out and that can be very disempowering for people who just want to get on with being a parent. You're working in partnership, and some (potential) foster carers just don't understand their role in the team.

And as Maisie goes on to say:

It's all so much harder than I ever imagined. I thought I was really sussed with children. I'd done a bit of co-parenting, had these relationships, been this spinster aunt, given advice. But it's so bloody different when you've got children here and so difficult when you have children whose backgrounds you don't know. So you don't know what's being triggered, and there's the whole relationship with Social Services. You've got a corporate parent coming in and just completely running the show, sometimes with corporate policies that seem nonsensical on an emotional level.

We also spoke to a very experienced foster carer, Pamela, who has two biological children of her own, has adopted ten children after having fostered them, and has fostered countless others. She still finds this aspect of fostering difficult:

With fostering, they're never yours and you have to ask permission for everything. If you want to do anything, you have to ring up Social Services and ask their permission. Quite rightly because I've been given responsibility to look after these children. But I've only ever got 90 per cent of it, there's always somebody, you know. If they need an operation, I've got to run around getting permission from Social Services whereas if they're your own children, you make that decision. That 10 per cent that is in other people's hands is hard to bear.

The rules can also make it difficult to act like a normal mum. Once they're a toddler, you can't have them in bed with you or in the bath. It's to protect you from any charge of abuse later, but it means you can't enjoy those intimate moments that are so precious to most mums.

While in some circumstances adoption may be an option, in the majority of cases foster caring is temporary and the child will move on. This could be particularly painful for a childless woman. Meryl Sturdy and her team are well aware of this, and try to support foster carers through this process:

We are really aware of the whole issue of loss for foster carers and how we support them. After a child has moved on we are very concerned that they have appropriate space to mourn the loss of that child and we would encourage a carer to keep her own life-story book, so she has a record of all the children she has cared for. And we would promote a foster carer staying in touch with the child, though we look at it from the child's point of view, so it must meet the child's needs.

As Maisie says about one of her two foster children, who has recently moved on:

I just had no idea that I'd kind of go into this 'Oh my God, where's my child gone?' It feels like I'm empty and I'm dead, and I hadn't expected to feel that. I'd done so much work with her and she's lovely, but she's hard work. I just went under, I kind of like went under emotionally, and I'm only just coming out of it now. I found it devastating; it felt just like a bereavement, it felt dreadful. I just hadn't realised how much it hurts when you have to let someone go. It's like when my sister's first born left home at the age of 24, she was in tears, she had a really tough time. But now she's looking forward to living out other bits of her life with her children, but in different ways. She was in the same boat as I was in around my child leaving, it was exactly the same, so I think it's just about individual connections to you and that child, and just the whole process of change and difference.

But Maisie certainly has no regrets about her decision to become a foster carer, and feels that she has gained a lot from the experience:

I know about children in a much more real sense, and I've learnt that I am a good enough parent and it's answered any questions I had about what sort of mother, what sort of parent I'd be. I would have liked the chance to have done it from scratch, but I trust I'm good enough. It's like becoming a member of that club. It's just so different being on the outside advising in and being that calm, cool, collected person that they can distress to and being the one who is pulling your hair out, realising how much it cost them, how much they really had to do, things you just couldn't have conceived of until you have those same worries and difficulties. It feels satisfying not to be wondering about all of the experience.

There are undoubtedly some particular challenges involved in foster caring and, if you are interested in exploring the possibility, there are details of who to contact in Appendix 1.

Relationships with children

Although initially, relationships with other people's children may be too painful, too immediate a reminder of our own loss, many of the women we spoke to gained great satisfaction from their involvement with children. For many of us, our relationships with nieces and nephews, or godchildren, or children of close friends, become much closer than they might have been, had we had our own children.

For Rebecca A, who is in her early 40s and single, it's her relationship with her brother's children that is important:

So I adopt, as it were, my brother's two children who I lavish my love upon. My love, my money – they are 10 and 6 – whenever possible they come and stay with me. They don't call me auntie, they call me Rebecca, which somehow makes it a closer relationship than an aunt and niece one. I am aware, and I hate to think I might one day burden them with my mismatched substitute mother role, I don't want it ever to become a burden for them, but that is what I'm doing. Most of the time, it's wonderful. I worry about them almost as much as if they were my own.

Habie has a very close relationship with her nieces and nephews, whom she refers to as her 'niblings':

I told my therapist at the IVF clinic yesterday that I went to see my sister in London and I played with the kids and then I came home on the train and I cried because I just borrowed her life for a day, and she's living the life I should have had. My therapist said 'But you didn't borrow her life, you are their aunt, that was your life.'

It really helped, because I suddenly thought 'Yes, I don't have to be a mum to love these kids.' My sister-in-law said to me 'You know, Hab, when you've got three kids and two full-time careers, you cannot give your kids full attention all the time.' She said 'I love it that when they're with you, you act as if they rule the world, as if nothing else in the day mattered, and you drop everything for them, and you listen to them.' She said 'It's lovely, because I know they're going to have a moment of pure indulgence.'

A few years ago, after having a miscarriage, Habie went to stay with her brother and his family. One morning, she was playing with her 2-year-old nephew:

It was very jolly, and he said to me 'This is my drill, my drill's bigger than daddy's drill', which I thought was like reading textbook Freud. Then he said 'I'm going to mend you because you're all broken.' And I hadn't said anything to him, not one thing, to him or in his hearing, but even though we were having fun and laughing he sensed that I was all broken, but that he could fix me, which was also true. Just being with him was fixing me.

Fay has a particularly close relationship with the family of her closest girlfriend:

It helps that this particular family see me as part of the family. My friend says that the children don't know that I'm not Auntie Fay; they think I'm part of the family, and I think I'm so lucky to have that contact. I have all the wonderful bits, and none of the difficult bits. This wonderful thing, of seeing the generation one down below me, so it would be, it's not my grandchildren, but as if it were, seeing them grow, seeing the development, seeing the excitement of being small children.

I suppose I sometimes think I'm a bit selfish about it, because I pop in and out as I can, so it's very nice, because I don't have the responsibility. I just feel I'm like, in a sense, the benign godparent for all of them, in that I'm outside of the family, but in the inner circle, or in the immediate circle of family, so can be someone that they could perhaps go to if they didn't want to go to the grandparents, or to mum or dad. I don't know. I'll see how it unfolds, really.

For many of us, our ability to enter into children's world without being a parent is a real bonus. We are able to have relationships with children that are based on choice and freedom, rather than duty.

For Helen, her relationship with her nephews is based on seeing them as little adults, and the emphasis is on having fun with them:

I enjoy spending time with my nephews. I enjoy the relationship that I have with them. I do see them as little people, I don't really see them as children; I just see them as small adults. I don't see them the way their mum sees them, really. We do loads of things, we're just utterly spontaneous, and you can be when you don't have children. I think their mum sometimes thinks that's really wonderful, even though I know she loves having the boys. To her, it's the old thing, familiarity, they're so every day to her, it's getting them up in the morning, getting them to school, making their lunches etc., and for me it's like I see them as little people. So I see some things, or notice things, or observe things that perhaps she doesn't always have the time or the energy to, and I really enjoy that, because I enjoy their differences.

Fay talked earlier about being a benign godparent to her closest friend's family. Here she talks about her relationship with the daughter of another friend:

One of my good friends died of cancer two years ago, and before she died her daughter had said to her 'You won't be around when I get married and come to buy a wedding dress.' My friend knew that I'm into clothes, and fashion, and said 'Fay's your woman.' She did this with each of her children, I think, made sure they had somebody that was for them, apart from godparents, and family, you know they've got all sorts of support.

But I just feel enormously privileged to have this young woman as a friend because she is an age that she could have been my daughter. I started out slightly thinking 'Ooh, that's nice, I've got a surrogate daughter', and then I realised that I didn't want a surrogate daughter, and that was a big realisation. She didn't need a surrogate mum, either, she had a mum. But I can be a special friend, and I just feel that's a huge privilege, to have a friend who's half my age. And she is a friend, it's wonderful, and I just think that's been very special. Perhaps if I'd got my own family I wouldn't have the time for that.

For Lucy B and her husband, not having their own children means they have more time to get involved with the children of their friends:

We do have a lot to do with children, with our friends' children, we're quite involved in their lives. It's different in that we have more time, we're not wrapped up in our own children, so we have more time to focus upon them, rather than be distracted. I think it gives both of us the pleasure of having children in your life, and we've seen some of our friends struggle with their children, things which cause them such worry, and such anxiety, that we're able to try and help them as outsiders.

Other forms of nurturing

Other people
Many of the women we spoke to found an outlet for their nurturing through their work.

Clare C is a complementary therapist, and is currently studying acupuncture:

[My maternal instinct] has come out in other ways, definitely, because of the work that I do. I've always been a bit touchy-feely and nurturing in my practice, I've given a lot to my patients over the years, and I've got lots of letters, cards, books that people have given me in appreciation of my care, so I've been very nurturing towards them. And actually doing this job at the moment, with the old folk, the little old lady that I was looking after last week was just like a baby, really. I loved taking care of her, because I could do my bit, which is what she needed. It's a heart thing, it's very female, very womanly, very physical, very much to do with warmth, and warm flesh, and hearts. She needed lots of cuddles, I need to cuddle.

Penny A teaches older teenagers, at a residential school:

Through my job I have a lot of contact with young people, which I enjoy. In some ways, there's a lot of parental aspect in teaching, I mean you're guiding them, I think I find that very satisfying. And actually, there's a lot of love in it as well. Obviously it's nothing like the love of a parent for a child, but it has elements of it. You see them develop, we had a graduation party last week and they left, you feel the same pride in how they've grown and the satisfaction they're moving on to the next stage of their life and so on, I enjoy that a lot.

And even if our jobs don't directly involve caring or teaching, many of us find opportunities for nurturing at work. Judy is a corporate vice-president with a major multinational organisation:

Over the years I developed really strong relationships with people a lot younger than me. And I have two of them, and they're like my little protégés, they're just wonderful. They joke about me being their mother; it's definitely that type of relationship, in that I really care about their well-being, what's going to happen to them. We're kind of peers and friends, but there's a lot of the mentoring type thing going on.

Fay works in organisational development:

The sort of work I've been doing until very recently has been around coaching people, about nurturing other people's skills, about helping people develop their relationships in a work environment, in a business environment, so perhaps I've put a lot of my nurturing into my work.

Many of the women we spoke to found an outlet for nurturing or mothering through voluntary work of various kinds: volunteering in a hospice, being a school governor, working for the Samaritans, being a school counsellor, becoming a prison visitor.

Linda is a lay magistrate, sitting in the Family Court, and she definitely sees this role as helping to satisfy her need to nurture:

Seeing how horrendous life could be for children, for so many children, I found it just soothing in a way that there were all these people out there with all these enormous problems who'd had all these children, and life was just unbearable. My great need to see these children settled somewhere, in a good home and looked after, was definitely part of that missing thing that I had.

It was soothing, in a way. I did feel like it was solving my problem as well as their problem. If I could sort this one out, if I could get this child away from this horrible situation and into a good one, then it was helping me to sort out my need to nurture more children. I was at least getting the children nurtured, maybe.

Lesley is a recovering alcoholic:

Having got sober, I did that by going to AA (Alcoholics Anonymous), and one of the things that happens on any of the 12-step fellowships is that you work your way through the 12 steps as a way of looking at the kind of patterns of thought and behaviour that have got you to where you are, and you ask somebody to help you do that. You then in turn help others. I have a number of people that I sponsor and take care of through that, and it's almost like I've been given a second chance at parenting, if you like, albeit with adults, but with people who've been through the same thing. I kind of think, well I can use my energy doing that, so I try to give back and pass on in an indirect way, through a different type of family, by doing that, and that has been a way of compensating for it.

Penny B has one daughter, but would have loved more. After deciding not to have any more IVF treatment, she and her husband got involved in a project organised at their local church:

What we did, which I threw myself into absolutely wholeheartedly, was have Chernobyl children, children from Byelorussia, every summer. What they do is they bring children who've been affected by the radiation over from Byelorussia once a year, and have them live with a host family in the summer. We had these two little girls over for the summer, and that was fantastic. I loved that, I loved being involved in the whole group thing, there were about 30 families and all the various kids, being involved in going off to different theme parks and taking the kids, and actually being involved on a one-to-one with the kids and looking after them, learning bits of Russian, the whole thing was just brilliant.

It was exhausting, absolutely exhausting but it fulfilled a need in me. The need to open our house to other children, on a sort of ... it wasn't fostering, but it was sort of looking after them for two weeks and getting to know them really well, but actually I felt I was doing something, the other side of fostering that I wanted to do, not just for me, but actually to give a child an experience of a home and living in a home, which I felt we could do, however imperfectly.

Janet and her husband sponsor a child in Africa:

We sponsor a boy in Sudan. My husband does a lot of work in developing countries, such as providing water solutions in Africa, India, Asia and things, so I think we would have always gone for that as a way of being charitable in a more direct fashion.

He writes to us and we write to him occasionally. It's a slow process because they have to clear everything, and he doesn't write that well, and I'm always hugely conscious of the richness that we have, the wealth we have, so it's hard to get the right balance in the conversation. There's a sort of nurturing side to it, we're interested in how he's doing at school and things. He wrote to us and said something about having to fetch water from the well and it's a long way away, so we're actually exploring whether we could sponsor a well in the village, so get involved more directly.

And if not through work, or voluntary work, many of us satisfy our need to nurture by having more time for our family and friends. Lesley talked above about sponsoring other people through AA. Her parents are both dead, and she only has distant relatives, all of whom live overseas:

I think there is a tendency to have a peer group who have not got children. I certainly have a close female grouping of women within ten years or so, and none of us have ever had children. For different reasons, actually. Within the recovery world people tend to have either had children a long time ago, and it's a complete fuck up, and they're scrabbling to try and put right the damage they've inflicted, or there's an awful lot of people, both male and female, who've never had them for very similar reasons.

You end up in something where, to a degree, you're parenting each other, and I have quite a strong network within that. For example, at the moment, one of my friends who is in a happy, long-term relationship with somebody, her mother, who is a sweetie, is, I think she's dying, actually. But there's a whole load of us who are all very much around, and are all very aware of what's going on and we're checking with each other, has anyone heard from her today, what's happened with her mum, and there's a kind of a family network that's developed around there. So I think you form virtual families.

Pets
There is no doubt that pets, like small babies, can fulfil our desire to give and receive unconditional love, and to have something that is totally dependent on us. Many of the women we spoke to talked

of their pets, albeit often with some embarrassment, as being surrogate children.

Rebecca B has been with her partner for seven years, and is a university lecturer:

I have cats. Such a stereotype. There's no question, I would have cats anyway, I love cats, but I do certainly put some of the feelings that I would put into children into my relationship with my cats. They're spoiled rotten. Obviously, there's a lot of things that you could give children ... you can't teach a cat, really. But I suppose just the affection, cuddles, calling them silly names and things. It's a kind of companionship too. I think the companionship that you can have with a small child and the companionship that you can have with an animal are quite similar, and very different from the kind of companionship that you have with another adult.

For Lesley, having a pet is about making a commitment:

I've nearly always had animals of some sort, mostly cats. If you're a non pet owner it sounds silly, but they are a commitment, and you can't have them and not have that kind of commitment, so there's that. They are surrogate kids, without a shadow of a doubt. Two very good friends of mine have got two cats and we actually laugh about it. We know each other very well, they will look after my cat, and we'll say, all three of us, we have our surrogates. We babysit, absolutely, yes, and you worry about them and do all of that, so there's that as well.

When Marti and her husband bought a house in the country, they also got a dog:

I don't think we realised how much we would love the dog when it came along. The reason I'm very upfront in saying that it's a child substitute is that I think there's no point in pretending otherwise. And I want him to have babies. We haven't had him done. We should have – he's a mongrel, for God's sake – and we haven't had him done because subconsciously, I think, we want to have a family with him.

Gardens and plants

It's interesting how many of the women we visited in the course of working on the book had beautifully tended gardens. When Clare A accepted that she was not going to have children, she took up gardening:

I took several vocational gardening courses. I noticed that a lot of people on the courses were people whose children had left home, sort of empty nesters, so I'd sort of basically skipped a stage, and apparently it's quite common for the nurturing side of people to come out in gardening. So a lot of the women that I met were turning that energy into their gardens, and learning about gardening. I found that quite helpful.

Françoise also talks about nurturing flowers, wondering whether really good gardeners aren't frustrated mothers. She recalls a time, almost 50 years ago:

I remember once when I was very depressed, after I'd had a miscarriage, in London. I put some seeds on the windowsill, and the pleasure it gave me when I suddenly saw them burgeoning, you know ...

Marti, who talked earlier about her dog being a child substitute, is also a keen gardener:

I've got a very big allotment, I grow my own vegetables, I love doing that. I do think that's part of a desire to create and grow and nurture and feed and do all that kind of thing. I'd much rather grow vegetables than flowers, or any of that stuff, I get a kick out of the fact that I can bring home all this fecundity, back to the house.

For many of us, the need or desire to nurture is strong, and it may well feel that we will not be able to fulfil this desire if we don't have children of our own. However, as we've seen in this chapter, many of the women we've talked to have successfully found alternative ways of fulfilling this desire.

CHAPTER 11

Alternative lifestyles

There are two key questions facing us, as childless women, 'Who am I, who will I be if not a mother?' and 'What will I do with the rest of my life?' There are no ready-made answers to these questions, and no obvious way to go about answering them. We all need to find our own road.

While trying to answer these questions can be very challenging, it can also represent a huge opportunity for us. Changing the focus from what we're not – a mother – to what we might be, can be frightening, but is also potentially very exciting. There may be few social conventions or templates to guide us, but then equally there are few to restrict us. We are back in control.

As Hilary Mantel writes, at the beginning of her memoir *Giving Up the Ghost*:

> *You come to this place, mid-life. You don't know how you got here, but suddenly you're staring fifty in the face. When you turn and look back down the years, you glimpse the ghosts of other lives you might have led. All your houses are haunted by the person you might have been. The wraiths and phantoms creep under your carpets and between the warp and weft of your curtains, they lurk in wardrobes and lie flat under drawer liners. You think of the children you might have had but didn't. When the midwife says 'It's a boy', where does the girl go? When you think you're pregnant and you're not, what happens to the child that has already formed in your mind? You keep it filed in a drawer of your*

consciousness, like a short story that wouldn't work after the opening lines.

I have hesitated for such a long time before beginning this narrative. For a long time I felt as if someone else were writing my life. I seemed able to create or interpret characters in fiction, but not able to create or interpret myself. About the time I reached mid-life, I began to understand why this was. The book of me was indeed being written by other people: by my parents, by the child I once was, and by my own unborn children, stretching out their ghost fingers to grab the pen. I began this writing in an attempt to seize the copyright in myself.

In terms of what we do with the rest of our lives, it's a fact that if we don't have dependants, we are probably more self-orientated than if we do. That doesn't necessarily make us selfish, and we don't need to beat ourselves up over it, but rather we can use that opportunity, that focus to find an alternative life to motherhood, one that brings us peace, happiness and fulfilment.

No one can answer these questions of identity and lifestyle for us, but in this chapter we'll hear from a number of women who've taken the first steps in attempting to seize the copyright in themselves and their lives.

Finding meaning and value

As we saw earlier, a sense of failure can be one of the key outcomes of wanting a child and not having one, and because of that, finding success in our lives can be very important. We've already seen how throwing ourselves into work is a common coping mechanism, but there are many other ways of finding achievement and fulfilment in our lives, and childlessness can be a trigger to re-evaluate what is important to us.

For me (Louise), it was the prospect of my 40th birthday, rather than my childlessness that led me to look again at my life and make some major changes. However, as I have already said, I used to joke that when I reached 40 I went from being too young to have children to being too old to have children overnight, so perhaps on some level, not consciously, I was accepting my childlessness and looking for a different path.

Two major realisations came to me. The first was that I was living the life of a married man, with a large house in the outer suburbs, commuting into the city every day to work. The only difference was that I didn't have a wife and children to come home to, like the other commuters I saw on the train every day. The second was, when I looked back at the first 20 years of my adult life, and my career, I felt pretty good about it: I'd been very successful, in material terms, and I had a strong sense of achievement and fulfilment from my work. However, when I looked forward and asked myself the question 'Do I want to spend the next 20 years doing more of the same?', the answer was a resounding 'No!'

I spent the next 18 months stumbling around in the dark, trying to figure out what to do: knowing what I didn't want was easy; working out what I did want was much harder. I started to put together a picture of what my life could be like – one where work would be a part of my life, rather than all-consuming, and one where I would have more time for other things and other people. On a holiday in Skyros (in fact, the same one where Rachel and I first met) I outlined my tentative thoughts to another guest. When I'd finished, he said 'So what's stopping you?'

It was the $64,000 question. It haunted me for months. It was difficult for me to accept, because I like to think of myself as a brave person, willing to take risks, but I finally realised that the only thing stopping me was fear.

I took a deep breath, and made the first tentative step by putting my house up for sale. I rationalised this by telling myself that it would probably take some time to sell my (rather unconventional) home, and that by moving I would immediately improve my quality of life, reducing my travelling time by two hours each day. Then, I thought, I could sit back and enjoy my new lifestyle, and work out what to do next.

Suddenly, everything happened very quickly – I found a buyer for the house straight away, moved into a rented flat, walking distance from my office, and a week after I moved saw an opportunity to negotiate redundancy from the company where I'd worked for 16 years. Six months after taking that first, tentative, step, I was without a house and without a job. I still didn't know what I wanted to do, but at least now I had the time and the space to explore. I decided to give myself at least two years before I worked again, to have some fun and figure out what to do next.

That was almost four years ago. I haven't worked since. For the first two years, I travelled, I sailed and I worked on my personal development, in centres in the UK, Greece, Spain and California. For the past two years, I've worked with Rachel on producing this book, something I would never have dreamt of in my previous life. I've had new experiences, and made lots of new friends. I still don't really know what I'm going to do in the longer term, but who does? I'm now much more interested in what's happening in the present.

Elisabeth is single and in her 40s, and has recently taken the decision to leave behind the world of advertising and retrain as a child psychotherapist:

I suppose I feel that I'm hopeful for myself that, even if I don't have children, I have finally found something that I really want to do, that actually means something to me. I've been working in a field where I've been thinking 'I'm not really part of this world, but I'm in it, I'm working in it.' I think that suited me quite well in a way, in that I could be in it, but feel detached at the same time. So I have a vision of myself, going into my 50s, as quite an interesting woman, with something to give, and I'll have got in touch with my creativity. I have a vision that I would love to write, and do things that I know I've had a longing to do and somehow my whole youth I've not allowed any of that to happen. The longing for a baby is part of that, but I'm beginning to long for things out of life and realise that life is there for the taking if I choose to grasp it.

Eve is a professional singer who, over the years, has gradually got her head around being childless:

To begin with, you just think 'What am I here for, what's the point?' But there is plenty of point. I just think the point in life is to get as much out of it as you can, and to try and put something back. Having a good relationship is very important, a relationship with your husband, with your friends, with your family, with people you work with.

As Fay goes through the menopause and the changes it brings, she reflects on her childlessness:

My body's maturing, and with that comes this realisation that I don't have the choice to have children any more, but perhaps I have many other things that have enabled me to feel part of [my closest friend's] family. Maybe it's just taught me that family comes in all sorts of different guises. It's the old truism that time does help. I think just realising that I have a very rich life. I don't mean rich in terms of money. I'm comfortably off, but it's not about that, it's the richness of friendships, it's the richness of feeling supported by people when I have needed it ... just feeling my place in the world in a very different way, and finding that place. It all sounds terribly grandiose, and I can't even tell you how it's happened, really.

Helen works in human resources, and has recently completed a Masters degree. She is currently taking a year's sabbatical to 'get back to basics' and decide what she wants from a job, and what she wants from her life:

I think the hardest part of being childless is how do you fulfil your life, and what's your life about. I think it's wrong to have children and think that is what fulfils your life, actually, I don't agree with that, but I think it's much easier. If you choose to lose yourself in that, you can. I think it's how do you find value in your life, how do you feel fulfilled, how do you feel like you're doing something of value, really, that's important.

I think you have to spend a lot of time thinking about what your talents are, what you're uniquely good at as an individual, and where your strengths are, and what you can do for other people. I do believe quite strongly that your relationships with other people are quite a big part of your value in life, in feeling fulfilled. I think if you can identify the ways in which you as an individual, what you're good at, what areas in your life you can do well in, you can give to other people, you can excel in – some of them might not be related to other people, you might be a fantastic artist or something. Again, it's perhaps back to this being content, finding what you're good at and being content with that, knowing 'This is what I am', not trying to be something that you're not, and doing what you can really well. Be good at doing what you can do.

As Deborah Vowles, MSc DipCouns, a counsellor who has worked on reproductive issues with couples with life-threatening illnesses and with conditions that might put a baby at risk, says:

If you haven't had children, you may feel you need to have your identity from something else, and not all of us do have brilliant careers. So where do we find a place to lodge an identity, a place to find an identity and a place to explore, nurture, express our creativity? If we can't create a baby, we can create a lovely garden or something, it's where do you find it.

Enjoying an unconventional lifestyle

Remaining childless may not have been our choice, but it can give us the opportunity to explore a whole range of options that might not otherwise have been open to us. We are fortunate, in that we have time, energy, money and flexibility that many of our peers who are parents just don't have.

For Clare B, who runs a ceramics workshop, not having children has ultimately been a very liberating experience:

The gains for me are about how I've discovered who I am and what I think is important in life. And the freedom to do whatever I feel I want to do – within reason, you have to earn a living. Things like my partner and I going off around the world for a year. We bought one of these round the world tickets, because we knew that once we set up the workshop we wouldn't have the time or money to do this trip. I'd always wanted to go and see Australia and New Zealand, and tour America, that sort of stuff, so we said 'Well let's just do it, we've got money', we both had our divorce monies through, 'Let's really just have a good time for a year and rejoice in the freedom and do what we want to do.'

I couldn't have done it [if I'd got children], I couldn't have gone away for a year and just left the children behind. And you couldn't travel like we did, taking them with you, because we were just sleeping in the car. We bought a car and slept in it, and that was how we lived, in various countries, we had different vehicles and bought and sold them. I know people do travel with children, but I don't think we could have done it like that. We couldn't have done it as we did it, literally making decisions from day to day on what we did, staying longer if we liked somewhere and leaving if we didn't. Because it was only us.

I think one of the reasons I really wanted to talk to you, when I heard what you were doing, because I wanted to share the fact that I'd actually found it very liberating, not to have children, having been quite upset to start with. So I felt quite strongly that I wanted to share that.

For me (Rachel), the second condition of my Survival Plan (see Chapter Five) was to have a lifestyle we couldn't possibly have if we had children. This was incredibly important for me; in the longer term, I needed to feel we were celebrating our childlessness, not continually mourning it.

After all the heartache, I relish the freedom of not having anyone or anything dependent on us. We have no set routines, we can do whatever we like, whenever we like – whether that's going to bed or getting up very early or very late, spending time together in remote, wild places, or for me, competing in triathlons and for my husband, racing cars or shooting. Nothing in our lives is fixed in stone. I love it, and I treasure the happiness and optimism I now feel, especially because it's been so hard earned. Trying my hand at new things, especially things that seem mad to everyone else, has been fantastic therapy in reinvigorating my life and making me feel proud of who I am.

When Sally and her husband stopped IVF, they moved house:

We were looking to move house, and we would not have been able to afford to buy that house if I had given up working, or was on part-time working if we weren't confident of the two incomes, but also knowing that we weren't looking for a family home whatever that means. There's a death trap for kids, if you had a toddler you just wouldn't, so moving into that house was immediately a decision, a kind of lifestyle thing in terms of this is going to be us on our own.

I would always have been drawn to an unconventional house, but I would have had to compromise if we'd had children, it would have been a happy compromise, so being drawn to that spectacular house, and being able to buy it felt good. I think at the time I was definitely on the search for projects, or a project that could help me look forward with some kind of joy and anticipation, so buying a house, moving in, doing it up was a project that felt positive. We just really liked the house, but we also knew that it would be fine for us living in it because we weren't looking for a house that would be good for children.

The thing that I really wanted, as a kind of consolation or compensation, was the fact that we did have the space, and the time, and the space in our lives to actually have room for friends, because of course people who have babies and small children are very wrapped up in that, they can't have lots of people to stay or do whatever. The house represented that as well.

For Liz and her partner, it's about things like the car they drive:

We do things like we have sports cars, we don't have estate cars. I think they're very sensible, because you can put the dog in the back, that's how I see an estate car. Our street is full of Mercedes estate cars, with Labradors and children in the back. Whereas we drive a two-door sports car, and all the kids in the street think it's really groovy. They think we're terribly cool because we've got this bright red sports car.

For Mary and her husband, being childless in the 1960s allowed them to have a much more adventurous lifestyle:

We started going abroad for holidays, in the 1960s. We were quite adventurous, in the 60s; 1962 we started to go abroad. It was the beginning of all the holiday brochures, they were suddenly appearing. There weren't that many travel agents about, you had to go looking; we went to a private one that was near to where we lived. [It made us feel] terrific, we were the smart set, weren't we? It felt great when you came back to work with this super tan, because we both go brown so easily.

The way I look at it, we've made a lifetime of memories that don't include children, but they were great, they're great memories. At my age now, when I had this heart bypass, you have to consider the possibility that you won't come out of it, but I wasn't scared because I thought how lucky I am to have got to this age and done everything I've done, and some poor people don't make it, do they? I think I've had a good life.

For Clare A, it's also about lifestyle:

[My lifestyle is] much more urban, the upside is that I'm much more culturally active and informed. Without wishing to sound snobby about this, I certainly know far more, I go far more to the new films, the new plays, the new restaurants than friends who possibly are living further out, or who are tied up and have babysitting worries. I think I probably get more out of the city because I'm free to do these things.

Exploring creativity

For many women, having children seems like the natural way to fulfil our desire to be creative. Habie, who is in her early 40s, has always wanted to write, and actually completed the first draft of a novel before everything else took second place to trying for a baby.

I always wanted to have the identity of a creative person, but I realised in the last five years that my creativity was to be a mother, and not having it has left me feeling like nothing. I tried to have babies, and you can't have babies and write novels at the same time, or at least my own personal emotional make up is like that. One creation at a time. And nothing will beat children, nothing beats making a human life.

Zoë Heller really put a spanner in my works by writing an article about how, when she had her two children in New York, she felt happy enough to really be a good writer. And sure enough, the book she's just written was shortlisted for the Booker prize, and this is with two small children, or one, and one on the way. And she said 'It was only when I had the happiness of my child that I was really able to write.' Whereas others have said you can only write when you haven't got kids, totally preoccupying, someone said 'The pram in the hall is the enemy of creativity' and I always believed I'd be so happy with my kids I could write even better.

Although it can be very difficult, a number of the women we have spoken to have found that being able to tap into their creativity, in ways other than producing children, has been a very fulfilling experience. As Dr Christiane Northrup says in her book *Women's Bodies, Women's Wisdom*:

> *We need to expand the meaning of fertility and birth. We must begin to see female birth power for what it is – the basis of all of creation. When enough women sense this creative female power inherent within each of us – not dependent on what we produce or don't produce with our bodies, not dependent on whom we let into our bodies – the world will change. When women tap into this power, the children, the ideas, and the new world to which we give birth will be supportive of all beings, including ourselves. Whether we ever choose pregnancy, every one of us has encoded in our cells the knowledge of what it is to conceive, gestate, and give birth to something that grows out of our own substance. You don't have to have a baby to learn how to labour. Labour, whether physical or metaphorical, teaches us not to fight the process of birthing, no matter what we're birthing, even when it hurts and we want to quit.*

After Lucy A had a hysterectomy in her late 30s, she decided to set up her own business sourcing and importing ceramics:

When I started my own company, that obviously took all my attention, and it became mine, I wasn't working for anybody else, everything I did was my own creation, all the selling was done the way I sell, all the flair came from me, the company's ethos came from me, came from my inside, so in a way that was one kind of channel. I know it's a different thing, but nonetheless it's something to channel your energies.

About eight years ago, Janet gave up her stressful, full-time consultancy role to become self-employed and to have more time for her pottery, which has gradually become her main occupation:

I think [the pottery is about] getting back to what I really am about, which is a creative person. It's taken me a while to have the confidence to do it, but I'm now selling my work professionally, but it's taken a long while to get to that confidence. It is about the core of me that got buried when academic achievement became important. I'm glad I did both, but I'm really glad that I found a way back to it, because I think a lot of people don't until it's too late, whereas at least I've done it now, in my 40s, when there's a chance to build a second sort-of career. I'm not sure how far I'll ever go with it, whether I'll become a famous potter or not, that sort of doesn't matter, it's just fulfilling in a different way.

Marilyn is a busy family doctor in her early 50s, and admits that she still has a slight niggle in the back of her mind that one day she and her husband might adopt. However, as she says:

I've started to think about all the other things I could do. Only recently. Studying philosophy, literature, courses, I ought to do a public speaking course, I can't public speak, I'd love to be able to sing, I'd like to arrange flowers ... it's about time I got on with life, I've been too busy working and now it's time to stop doing that and do all these other things, which are really quite productive and fun. They're all quite artistic, nurturing. I don't think I need to build a house just to put children in, I think I need to build a house because I want to build a house.

Making a contribution

We have seen already that for many of us wanting a child is linked to reaching that stage in our lives where we want to give something to someone else, not just to our partner and our relatives, to put something back, to interact with the wider community and the wider world. This desire isn't confined to the childless, but those of us without children are superbly placed to do something about it, and the women we have spoken to have channelled this desire in a variety of ways.

For us (Rachel and Louise), the motivation for writing this book was definitely about reaching out to the community of childless women, creating something that didn't exist, leaving our legacy – this book is definitely our 'baby'! And many of the women we spoke to spontaneously expressed their satisfaction at being able to contribute to something that would help other childless women.

Similarly, Eve, who talked earlier about the importance of relationships, feels good about being able to use her own experience to help a girlfriend in a similar situation:

There's one girlfriend that I did talk to a lot about it to begin with. Now she's in a situation, she's 37 and she's going out with a guy who's just turned 30 and is not awfully keen on settling down. Of course she realises that time is marching on, and she's the one who now tries to broach the subject with me about the possibility that she might not ever have any children, and how do you get your head around it, kind of thing. That's quite interesting, to be able to give words of wisdom to somebody else. It makes me feel quite good, because I think 'Well actually, yes, I can help somebody else with it, I'm not the one that needs to be helped any more.'

Paula is currently caring full time for her elderly mother. She reflects on what she might do in the future:

My dream is to help people, because there's so much agony in the world that you've got to be able to help. In a way I feel that it's probably a good thing that I don't have children, because then I won't be dragged back, thinking I've got to look after them and be there for them. At least I'm free to do that. This is why I love this space; it doesn't make me claustrophobic. I just love a big, wide open space, to be free. I need freedom to paint, to feel free in myself and to help other people.

Heather sees one of the gains of her childlessness as being able to make a contribution, and take risks, in a way that would not otherwise have been possible:

The gain is my independence, my ability to do whatever I want, whenever I want to do it. And actually, the gain has been some of the voluntary stuff I've done, I've been to places in the world, I've done things that I would never, ever have done if I'd had children. I've worked with refugees in camps in Sudan and Egypt, in quite dangerous situations, been held up at gunpoint in Somalia and I would never have put myself in that position ... I put myself in that position because at the end of the day, there's only me, really, to worry about. I mean people would be very sad if I was killed but there's no one dependent on me, you take responsibility.

Janet, who talked earlier about becoming a professional potter, is also very involved in her local community:

I'm running a lot of nurturing type things in the village. I've set up two children's groups in the village to give the youngsters other outlets for developing. Plus I chair, I run the village fete, and I run a local society which is about preserving our local history and landscape and things like that. I'm quite green in my politics if anything, so it's all about environmental stuff too.

I think it's the bit I could have given to children I'm now giving to the community. I do a lot of leadership in the village. All I've done is transfer my corporate skills to a village environment, in some ways. I just passionately believe, I suppose, that community matters and that people belonging to each other is really important, and that we need to support communities in different ways. That's a large part of what I do, making sure that the community that I've joined stays a community. It's preservation, I guess, because you see so much disintegration, people being so isolated, it seems such a shame.

Building a new identity and a new lifestyle

I (Rachel) came across a thought in one of those self-help books I can never resist, which said 'There is no single reality, just your current model of it. If you don't like your reality, change it.' I keep it stuck on the wall next to my PC as I find it very useful in helping me jettison my negative image of myself as a non-mother. I'm slowly beginning to see myself, and to enjoy seeing myself, as a woman in my own right, free of dependants, and together with my husband being able to take advantage of whatever opportunities come our way. I know there will be times ahead when I'll feel the pain of my childlessness again, but I've come to accept this as recognition of my loss. I see myself as a survivor of childlessness and I'm proud of that achievement. I've come a very long way from that night in the chalet in Zermatt.

As Alison Bagshawe, Senior Fertility Counsellor at Guy's Hospital, says:

Many women face the issues of 'Who am I? What do I do? Where do I go?' at 50, or whenever their children grown up, and they don't know. I think if you face that earlier, for example through childlessness, you've actually got the world at your feet, you've got more chance to develop your full potential. If you can turn it round, you can create something, and become what you're meant to be. This is such a generalisation, but certainly friends, people I know, their lives rotate around children, until the children are 20 or even 30. I think that they're so busy, their life is so financially wrapped up, so emotionally wrapped up and so physically wrapped up in their children's lives, that many never fulfil their own potential. There is a light at the end of the tunnel, and there are ways of moving out of this. It's not the be all and end all, and although it feels it at the time, it isn't.

As we said at the beginning of this chapter, it's not easy facing up to the questions 'Who am I, who will I be if not a mother?' and 'What will I do with the rest of my life?'. We certainly don't claim to have ready-made answers, and neither would any of the women we talked to. But we sincerely hope that their stories will inspire you, as they have us, with a sense of the range of possibilities that is open to all of us, and the knowledge that there can be life beyond childlessness.

Postscript: 'Do you have children?'

We started this book with our own answers to the question 'Do you have children?' In our view, how you answer this question, and how you feel about your response, can tell you a lot about where you are on your journey of learning to live with childlessness.

Here are just a few examples from the women we talked to:

I'll say 'No, I don't actually', and I'll feel a bit 'less than'. I will feel like that I haven't done something that was kind of expected of me ... It's funny, isn't it, expected of me, I wonder where that came from? I haven't quite conformed somehow, is part of that, but also I've been a bit of a let down, it feels like. To whom, I don't know. (Lesley)

I usually just say 'No', rather than 'Not yet', or whatever, and I have to say, I always feel slightly awkward. I suppose the reason I feel awkward is that I would love to be able to launch into the whole 'I would really like to but my partner doesn't', but you can't go around laying all that stuff on somebody that you've only just met. It's partly just English reserve, I suppose, but also I suppose I wouldn't want someone that I didn't know very well to feel that I was blaming my partner for something that I'm unhappy about, which in a way I do, I suppose, but I don't exactly feel I ought to, if you know what I mean. (Rebecca B)

I've just come back from a holiday and the inevitable question, wherever you are in the world, is always 'How many children do you have?' There is an expectation that you will have children. This was South

America, but it happens almost everywhere, except possibly the States. So you say 'Well, none', and then there's this horrified silence, when nobody knows what to say. And I never know how to fill it. You'd think after all this time I would have actually come up with a better answer than 'None', and I must work on that.

I now do it by saying 'Well actually, I don't have any, do you?' And I always just throw it back, and they generally do [have children] because actually if you don't have children, you don't tend to ask. So they'll always come back with an answer, and I just deflect it away, is actually what I do. (Heather)

I say 'No, I have a dog', and immediately get out photographs of him to show them. (Marti)

I usually say 'Not that I know of.' I like the way men say that, very smarmily, I like the idea that perhaps I could have had gestation and popped a baby out without even noticing it. I suppose it's because I don't want to be pitied. (Maria)

I say 'No, I've got two stepchildren.' Because people then assume that maybe you didn't want to have children, and your husband already had children. There are all sorts of other issues that one assumes people are thinking about, which they're probably not, like 'Oh yes, well she probably married someone who'd been married and had a vasectomy and had these two children.' So I feel there's much less instantaneous judgement of me. (Marilyn)

I always tell people 'I haven't got children because I can't have them.' I don't want people thinking that I have chosen not to. It's really important to me that people know that I haven't chosen. (Anne B)

In fact, since writing the book I (Louise) have now changed my response. In appropriate circumstances, I will now say 'No. I would have liked to, but I was never in the right relationship at the right time.' That feels good. It feels true to myself, and I no longer worry about what the person asking the question might be thinking.

Other women have found that deciding to change their answer to this question can be another positive step on their journey.

I've got better, I've got calmer. I usually say 'Unfortunately, I don't.' When I was on a study visit last Easter a woman who was getting decidedly drunk said 'Oh aren't you lucky.' I was leading the trip, so I was supposed to remain professional, but with tears welling up in my eyes, I said 'No, I regard myself as very unlucky.' She was too drunk to notice or care, but it was a big step for me to actually say that publicly. (Rebecca A)

I just say 'No, I don't.' I used to say 'Unfortunately no, I haven't', but now I just say 'No, I don't.' I can't be bothered explaining to people about it if they ask, I just think 'Here we go again.' And I think just because I feel more positive in it now, that I don't feel I need to, I don't feel I want to say 'No, I haven't', in a sad way, I just say 'No, I don't', in a matter of fact way. I felt I gave that [sad] response because I wanted people to feel sorry for me, and I wanted people to say 'Oh how terrible for you', and 'What happened?'

It makes me feel quite good, actually, I think because it reinforces the fact that it's not an issue for me so much now. It's kind of a little next step forward. Not that I ever plotted out a path that I had to follow for it or anything, but it makes me feel happy because I feel confident to say that, to give that answer, and to feel good about giving that answer, and I don't feel that I'm telling an untruth by giving that answer. (Eve)

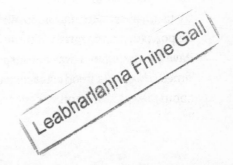

Practical support

This section contains contact details for a variety of organisations that may be helpful for readers of *Beyond Childlessness*. While we have tried to ensure, as far as possible, that we have only included reputable and responsible organisations, the inclusion of any organisation in this list does not represent any endorsement by the authors.

Reproductive health

MoreToLife

Charter House, 43 St Leonards Road, Bexhill-on-Sea, East Sussex TN40 1JA

Tel: +44 (0) 8701 188088 Website: www.infertilitynetworkuk.com

A national organisation, part of Infertility Network UK, dedicated solely to providing support to individuals and couples who, involuntarily, remain child-less. The service offers a lending library of useful books, factsheets, newsletters and a network of members throughout the UK, some of whom link up in person or by telephone to offer mutual support.

ARC, Antenatal Results and Choices

73–75 Charlotte Street, London W1P 4PN

Tel: +44 (0) 20 7631 0285 Website: www.arc-uk.org

Non-directive information and support for parents throughout the antenatal testing process and when an abnormality is diagnosed in their unborn child.

Daisy Network

PO Box 183, Rossendale BB4 6WZ

Website: www.daisynetwork.org.uk

National charity and support group for women suffering from premature menopause; that is before the age of 40.

Endometriosis SHE Trust (UK)

14 Moorland Way, Lincoln LN6 7JW

Tel: +44 (0) 8707 743664 Website: www.shetrust.org.uk

National charity offering help, holistic information and support to women with endometriosis to be able to make informed choices about conventional, nutritional and complementary therapies.

The Human Fertilisation and Embryology Authority

21 Bloomsbury Street, London WC1B 3HF

Tel: +44 (0) 20 7291 8200 Website: www.hfea.gov.uk

Non-departmental government body regulating all UK fertility clinics and a useful source of information and publications on all aspects of fertility treatment.

Infertility Network (IN) UK

Charter House, 43 St Leonards Road, Bexhill-on-Sea, East Sussex TN40 1JA

Tel: +44 (0) 8701 188088 Website: www.infertilitynetworkuk.com

National charity created by merger of CHILD and ISSUE, providing advice, support and understanding for those experiencing fertility problems.

The Menopause Amarant Trust

Tel: (+44 (0) 1293 413000 Website: www.amarantmenopausetrust.com

Aims to help women deal with problems they might experience while going through the menopause.

The National Endometriosis Society

50 Westminster Palace Gardens, Artillery Row, London SW1P 1RR

Tel: +44 (0) 20 7222 2781 Website: www.endo.org.uk

Self-help group for women with endometriosis.

National Infertility Awareness Campaign (NIAC)

NIAC PO Box 2106, London W1A 3DZ

Tel: +44 (0) 800 716345 Website: www.repromed.co.uk/niac/

A voluntary organisation campaigning for better provision of infertility treatment services on the NHS. The campaign includes awareness roadshows, briefings to MPs and an annual Infertility Focus Week, usually in June.

WellBeing of Women

27 Sussex Place, Regents Park, London NW1 4SP

Tel: +44 (0) 20 7772 6400 Website: www.wellbeing.org.uk

Funds research into all aspects of women's reproductive health and provides information leaflets on a wide range of issues from infertility to coping with pregnancy loss through miscarriage, stillbirth or newborn death.

Women's Health

52 Featherstone Street, London EC1Y 8RT

Tel: +44 (0) 20 7251 6333 Website: www.womenshealthlondon.org.uk

National voluntary independent organisation providing health information on a wide range of gynaecological health issues, together with booklets, a helpline and self-help support network.

Alternative parenting

Adoption

Adoption UK

46 The Green, South Bar Street, Banbury OX16 9AB

Tel: +44 (0) 1295 752240 Website: www.adoptionuk.com

National self-help group run by adoptive parents providing support, friendship and information to adoptive parents and prospective adopters before, during and after adoption.

British Association for Adoption and Fostering (BAAF)

Skyline House, 200 Union Street, London SE1 0LX

Tel: +44 (0) 20 7953 2000 Website: www.baaf.org.uk

Sets standards, raises awareness, influences policy and assists agencies across the UK to find permanent families for children separated from their birth families.

Coram Family

Coram Community Campus, 49 Mecklenburgh Square, London WC1N 2QA

Tel: +44 (0) 20 7520 0300 Website: www.coram.org.uk

A children's charity for the care of vulnerable children and their families. Services include fostering and adoption.

Overseas Adoption Helpline

64-66 High Street, Barnes, Herts EN5 5SJ

Tel: +44 (0) 870 516 8742 Website: www.oah.org.uk

A charity providing independent, accurate information and advice for anyone in the UK who is considering adopting a child from abroad.

Fostering

The Fostering Network

Tel: +44 (0) 20 7261 1884 Website: www.thefostering.net

UK's leading charity for everyone involved in fostering. The site includes information on becoming a foster carer and a directory to locate your local fostering service.

Surrogacy

COTS (Childlessness Overcome Through Surrogacy)

Lairg, Sutherland IV27 4EF

Tel: +44 (0) 844 414 0181 Website: www.surrogacy.org.uk

A voluntary organisation providing advice, help and support to surrogates and intended parents within the UK.

Surrogacy UK

PO Box 24, Newent, GL18 1YS

Tel: +44 (0) 1531 821889 Website: www.surrogacyuk.org

Provides help, advice and support to surrogates and intended parents within the UK.

Loss and bereavement

The Foundation for the Study of Infant Deaths

Artillery House, 11-19 Artillery Row, London SW1P 1RT

Tel: +44 (0) 870 787 0554 Website: www.sids.org.uk

UK's leading cot death charity funds research, supports bereaved families and disseminates information about cot deaths and baby care.

Meredith Wheeler

St. Martin de Dauzats, Lautrec, 81440 France

Tel: +33 563 59 11 32 Email: meredith.wheeler@free.fr

A transpersonal psychotherapist who runs workshops in the UK on letting go and coming to terms with loss experienced around involuntary childlessness, whatever the circumstances.

The Miscarriage Association

c/o Clayton Hospital, Northgate, Wakefield WF1 3JS

Tel: +44 (0)1924 200799 Website: www.miscarriageassociation.org.uk

Provides support and information after miscarriage.

SANDS, The Stillbirth and Neonatal Death Society

28 Portland Place, London W1B 1LY

Tel: +44 (0) 20 7436 5881 Website: www.uk-sands.org

Provides support for parents and families whose baby is stillborn or dies soon after birth.

Counselling

If you are considering counselling, it is important to spend time finding someone whose training and experience best suits your needs. Initially, it may be advisable to approach your family doctor. Many medical practices now have a resident counsellor, psychologist and/or psychotherapist and all practices run a referral service.

British Association for Counselling and Psychotherapy (BACP)
BACP House, 35-37 Albert Street, Rugby, Warwickshire CV21 2SG
Tel: +44 (0) 870 443 5252 Website: www.counselling.co.uk
National charity providing information on counselling and psychotherapy with a directory of therapists.

British Association for Sexual and Relationship Therapy (BASRT)
PO Box 13686, London SW20 9ZH
Tel: +44 (0) 20 8543 2707 Website: www.basrt.org.uk
National specialist charity maintains a list of accredited therapists and also sets standards and provides training/education for therapists and clinicians. Promotes research and provides information on sexual problems.

British Confederation of Psychotherapists (BCP)
West Hill House, 6 Swains Lane, London N6 6QS
Tel: +44 (0) 20 7267 3626 Website: www.bcp.org.uk
An association, linking societies offering psychotherapy and psychoanalysis, offering an on-line register of therapists, which is also available by post.

British Infertility Counselling Association
69 Division Street, Sheffield S1 4GE
Tel: +44 (0) 114 263 1448 Website: www.bica.net
Advises on how best to choose a counsellor and has a list of accredited infertility counsellors.

Choosing Talking Therapies?

DH Publications, PO Box 777, London SE1 6XH

Email: doh@prolog.uk.com

A free Government booklet explaining what talking therapies are and what they aim to do, helping you ask the right questions and make the right choices. To receive the booklet write to the address above.

Couple Counselling Scotland

Locate nearest branch on-line or via telephone directory

Website: www.couplecounselling.org

Formerly Marriage Counselling Scotland, a charity with local branches across Scotland offering counselling for couples irrespective of status and sexuality.

Relate

Central office: Herbert Gray College, Little Church Street, Rugby CV21 3AP

Tel: +44 (0) 845 456 1310 Website: www.relate.org.uk

Offers advice, relationship counselling and sex therapy face-to-face, by phone or online.

UK Council for Psychotherapy (UKCP)

167-169 Great Portland Street, London W1W 5PF

Tel: +44 (0) 20 7436 3002 Website: www.psychotherapy.org.uk

The council has a register of experienced psychotherapists for the exploration of difficult and often painful emotions and experiences.

Women's Therapy Centre

10 Manor Gardens, London N7 6JS

Tel: +44 (0) 20 7263 6200 Website: www.womenstherapycentre.co.uk

Provides subsidised low-cost psychotherapy on a sliding scale for women by women plus a referral service for those seeking a psychotherapist in private practice.

Agencies outside the UK

European Infertility Network

Website: www.ein.org

A worldwide infertility site providing information, books and CDs on assisted reproduction.

Honored Babies

Website: www.honoredbabies.org

An online women's support group offering a safe place to share feelings, experiences and memorials for the loss of a baby through miscarriage, ectopic pregnancy, termination, stillbirth, neonatal and infant death.

iCSi International Consumer Support for Infertility

Website: www.icsi.ws

A patient leader network established to empower patients to become full partners in ART (fertility) healthcare and public policy by building effective relationships with providers, governments and media worldwide. The organisation produces fact sheets on all aspects of infertility.

Perspectives Press

Website: www.perspectivespress.com

An American infertility and adoption publisher producing books, articles, seminars, workshops on infertility, reproductive health and alternative family building – from adoption to collaborative reproduction to fostering to childfree living.

Australia and New Zealand

ACCESS Australia's National Infertility Network

PO Box 959, Parramatta NSW 2124, Australia

Tel: +61 (0) 2 9670 2380 Website: www.access.org.au

An independent, non-profit organisation providing information, fact sheets, contacts for those sharing a particular infertility treatment, regular newsletter, register of self- help groups, infertility counsellors and accredited fertility clinics.

AFC Australian Families for Children
PO Box 7420, Bondi Beach NSW 2026, Australia
Tel: +61 (0) 2 9371 9244 Website: www.australiansadopt.org
Dedicated to finding permanent families in Australia for overseas children who have no possibility of family life in their country of birth.

AISG Australian Infertility Support Group
Website: www.nor.com.au/community/AISG
An internet-based support group for people living in Australia and New Zealand sharing knowledge, resources and support for those dealing with infertility, considering adoption or childfree living.

The Australasian Menopause Society
PO Box 12228, Buderin, Queensland 4556, Australia
Tel: +61 (0) 7 5456 2660 Website: www.menopause.org.au
Information, advice and support on the menopause for women in Australia and New Zealand.

Fertility NZ
PO Box 34 151, Birkenhead, Auckland, New Zealand
Tel: +61 (0) 800 333 306 Website: www.fertilitynz.org.nz
Voluntary organisation established by infertile people, with branches across New Zealand, to support, guide, provide information, educate and advocate on all aspects of infertility and its treatment.

ICANZ Inter Country Adoption New Zealand
PO Box 96-124, Balmoral, Auckland, New Zealand
Tel: +64 (0) 9 623 9369 Website: www.icanz.gen.nz
Helping New Zealanders adopt internationally, an holistic approach assisting adoptive families, before, during and after the adoption.

Miscarriage Support Auckland Inc
PO Box 14 7011 Ponsonby, Auckland, New Zealand
Website: www.miscarriagesupport.org.nz
Branches nationwide of volunteers, all of whom have lost babies, offering emotional and psychological support and information to women and their families during and after miscarriage, or as they prefer to call it, premature stillbirth.

NZEF New Zealand Endometriosis Foundation
In person: Suite 75, Blackheath, 75 Durham Street, Christchurch
Mail to: PO Box 1673, Mail Centre, Christchurch
Tel: +61 (0) 3 379 7959 Website: www.nzendo.co.nz
Providing information, education and encouraging research to support women,
girls and families living with endometriosis.

PACFA, Psychotherapy and Counselling Federation of Australia
P.O. Box 481, Carlton South, Vic 3053
Tel: +61 (0) 9639 8330 Website: www.pacfa.org.au
Information on different types of therapy together with a national register of
accredited therapists.

South Africa
Family and Marriage Society of South Africa (FAMSA)
Mail: PO Box 2800, Kempton Park 1620, South Africa
In Person: 15 Pascoe Avenue, Kempton Park, South Africa
Tel: +27 (0) 11 975 7107 Website: www.famsa.org.za
A non-profit countrywide network of societies established to help empower people
to build, reconstruct and maintain sound relationships in marriages, families
and communities, offering, among other services, specialist counselling for indi-
viduals, couples and families.

USA
American Fertility Association
666 5th Avenue, Suite 278, New York, NY 10103-0004
Tel: +1 888 917 3777 Website: www.theafa.org
A national American, non-profit organisation serving the unique needs of men
and women confronting infertility issues including helping couples make
informed decisions throughout the infertility process and informing on all forms
of family building.

Joint Council on International Children's Services
117 South Saint Asaph Street, Alexandria, VA 22314
Tel: +1 703 535 8045 Website: www.jcics.org/international_adoption.htm
An American site giving information and advice on inter-country adoption.

Resolve, The National Infertility Association

Tel: +1 888 623 0744 Website: www.resolve.org

Established in 1974, the organisation is dedicated to providing education, advocacy and support for men and women facing the crisis of infertility, and includes information on adoption and living childfree.

SHARE, Pregnancy and Infant Loss Support Inc

St Joseph Health Center, 300 First Capitol Drive, St Charles, Missouri 63301-2893

Tel: +1 800 821 6819 Website: www.nationalshareoffice.com

A national not-for-profit non-denominational organisation with over 130 chapters providing emotional, physical, spiritual and social support to those whose lives are touched by the tragic death of a baby through early pregnancy loss, stillbirth or newborn death.

Personal development

Personal development is a vast area, and the organisations detailed below are a small selection, of which the authors have had some personal experience. While these organisations have helped us in our search for identity and lifestyle, they may or may not be right for you.

Within the UK

Alternatives

St. James's Church, 197 Piccadilly, London W1J 9LL

Tel: +44 (0) 20 7287 6711 Website: www.alternatives.org.uk

A non-profit making, non-religious organisation dedicated to the exploration of different ways of living and being, through a diverse programme of talks and workshops.

The Essence Foundation

Lonsto House, Princes Lane, London N10 3LU

Tel: +44 (0) 20 8883 2888 Website: www.essence-foundation.com

A not-for-profit organisation running courses allowing people to take steps inside themselves to achieve personal power, freedom and a better quality of life.

Fiona Harrold Consultancy

71a Lysia Street, London SW6 6NF

Tel: +44 (0) 845 095 5541 Website: www.fionaharrold.com

An inspirational life coach and author who, with her life coaching team, gives talks and runs workshops and courses on personal development, both in person and online, as well as offering one-to-one life coaching. You can also subscribe to a free weekly online newsletter.

The Gestalt Centre

62 Paul Street, London EC2A 4NA

Tel: +44 (0) 20 7613 4480 Website: www.gestaltcentre.co.uk

A not-for-profit company that runs free open evenings explaining the gestalt approach and their programme of experiential groups and training courses. The Centre also runs a client referral service for those seeking counselling or therapy.

Outside the UK

Cortijo Romero

22 Cottage Offices, Latimer Park, Latimer, Chesham HP5 1TU

Tel: +44 (0) 1494 765775 Website: www.cortijo-romero.co.uk

Year-round alternative holidays in Andalucia, Spain offering a wide range of personal development courses and workshops.

The Esalen Institute

55000 Highway 1, Big Sur, CA 93920-9616, USA

Tel: 001 831 667 3000 Website: www.esalen.org

A California-based alternative educational centre devoted to the exploration of human potential. It offers workshops ranging from weekends to long-stay residencies.

Feminenza

PO Box 271, Welwyn Garden City AL7 1WJ

Tel: +44 (0) 1707 335 420 Website: www.feminenza.org

A worldwide women's group running workshops, courses and talks in the UK and internationally, based on the belief that women need to know themselves better, find their inner strength and a connection to the deepest parts of themselves to be able to fully play their part in the future of the world.

Neal's Yard Agency
BCM Neal's Yard, London WC1N 3XX
Tel: +44 (0) 870 444 2702 Website: www.nealsyardagency.com
A leading source of information on courses, retreats, wellbeing holidays and short breaks – the worldwide travel agent for inner journeys.

The Red Hat Society
Website: www.redhatsociety.com
An organisation of women united in celebrating life over 50, also open to younger women. Originating in the US, it now has chapters all over the world, including the UK, South Africa, Australia and New Zealand.

Skyros Holistic Holidays
92 Prince of Wales Road, London NW5 3NE
Tel: +44 (0) 20 7267 4424 Website: www.skyros.com
Holidays based at centres in Greece and Thailand offering a wide range of courses including writing, alternative therapies, arts and crafts and personal development.

APPENDIX 2

Bibliography

Recommended reading

Carter, Jean W. and Carter, Michael (1998) *Sweet Grapes: How to Stop Being Infertile and Start Living Again.* Perspectives

Edelman, Hope (1994) *Motherless Daughters – The Legacy of Loss.* Dell Publishing

Hewlett, Sylvia Ann (2002) *Baby Hunger – The New Battle for Motherhood.* Atlantic Books

Ironside, Virginia (1997) *You'll Get Over It – The Rage of Bereavement.* Penguin

Mantel, Hilary (2003) *Giving Up the Ghost – a Memoir.* Fourth Estate

Remen, Rachel Naomi (1996) *Kitchen Table Wisdom: Stories That Heal.* Riverhead Books

Sheehy, Gail (1997) *New Passages – Mapping Your Life Across Time.* HarperCollins

Welshons, John E. (2003) *Awakening from Grief – Finding the Way Back to Joy.* Inner Ocean Publishing

Other reading

Alden, Paulette Bates (1998) *Crossing the Moon – A Woman's Struggle to Have a Child Yields a Joyful Surprise – the Birth of a New Self.* Penguin

Anton, Linda Hunt (1992) *Never to be a Mother – A Guide for All Women who Didn't – or Couldn't – Have Children.* HarperSanFrancisco

Armstrong, Pamela (1996) *Beating the Biological Clock – The Joys and Challenges of Late Motherhood.* Headline

Bennett, Alan (2004) *The History Boys.* Faber and Faber

Berryman, Julia; Thorpe, Karen and Windridge, Kate (1995) *Older Mothers: Conception, Pregnancy and Birth after 35.* Pandora

Biggs, Sarah (2000) *Considering Adoption.* Sheldon Press

Brady, Joan (1998) *I Don't Need a Baby to Be Who I Am.* Pocket Books

Brian, Kate (1998) *In Pursuit of Parenthood – Real Life Experiences of IVF.* Bloomsbury

Brown, Helen Gurley (1982) *Having It All.* Simon & Schuster

Bryan, Elizabeth and Higgins, Ronald (1995) *Infertility: New Choices, New Dilemmas.* Penguin

Carlson, Richard, PhD (2002) *What About the Big Stuff? Finding strength and Moving Forward When the Stakes are High.* Hodder & Stoughton

Casey, Terri (1998) *Pride and Joy – The Lives and Passions of Women Without Children.* Beyond Words Publishing Inc.

DeFrain, John; Ernst, Linda; Jakub, Deanne and Taylor, Jacque (1991) *Sudden Infant Death – Enduring the Loss.* Lexington

Field, Lynda (2001) *Just Do it Now – How to Become the Person You Most Want to Be.* Vermilion

Francis-Cheung, Theresa (2001) *Cope with your Biological Clock – How to Make the Right Decision About Motherhood.* Hodder & Stoughton

Fraser, Ginny (2001) *A Mother in my Heart – How to Overcome the Pain of Involuntary Childlessness.* Nightlight Publishing

Friedan, Betty (1993) *The Fountain of Age.* Random House

Goldstein, Dr Andrew and Brandon, Dr Marianne (2004) *Reclaiming Desire: A Guide to Finding Your Lost Libido.* Rodale

Haynes, Jane and Miller, Juliet (ed.) (2003) *Inconceivable Conceptions – Psychological Aspects of Infertility and Reproductive Technology.* Brunner-Routledge

Houghton, Diane and Houghton, Peter (1984) *Coping with Childlessness.* Allen & Unwin

Ironside, Virginia and Biggs, Sarah (1995) *The Subfertility Handbook.* Sheldon Press

James, Oliver (2002) *They F**k You Up – How to Survive Family Life.* Bloomsbury

Kluger-Bell, Kim (1999) *Unspeakable Losses – Understanding the Experience of Pregnancy Loss, Miscarriage and Abortion.* Penguin

Kohner, Nancy and Henley, Alix (2001) *When a Baby Dies – The Experience of Late Miscarriage, Stillbirth and Neonatal Death*. Routledge

Lafayette, Leslie (1995) *Why Don't You Have Kids? Living a Full Life Without Parenthood*. Kensington

Lang, Susan S. (1991) *Women without Children – The Reason, the Rewards, the Regrets*. Pharos

Lisle, Laurie (1999) *Without Child – Challenging the Stigma of Childlessness*. Routledge

Love, Vicky (1984) *Childless is Not Less*. Bethany House

Montgomery, Bob and Morris, Dr Laurel (1989) *Surviving – Coping With a Life Crisis*. Lothian

Northrup, Christiane MD (2002) *Women's Bodies, Women's Wisdom – Creating Physical and Emotional Health and Healing*. Bantam

Ratner, Rochelle (ed.) (2001) *Bearing Life – Women's Writing on Childlessness*. Feminist Press

Rehner, Jan (1989) *Infertility – Old Myths, New Meanings*. Second Story Press

Ryan, Regina Sara (1993) *No Child in My Life*. Stillpoint

Safer, Jeanne (1996) *Beyond Motherhood – Choosing a Life Without Children*. Pocket Books

Tatelbaum, Judy (1997) *The Courage to Grieve – Creative Living, Recovery and Growth Through Grief*. Vermilion

Taylor Fleming, Anne (1994) *Motherhood Deferred – A Woman's Journey*. Putnams NY

Taylor, Laurie and Taylor, Matthew (2003) *What are Children For?* Short Books

Trevelyan, Joanna (1998) *But I Want a Baby – Infertility, Your Options*. Headline

Winston, Professor Robert (1999) *The IVF Revolution – The Definitive Guide to Assisted Reproductive Techniques*. Vermilion

Index

OTHER RODALE BOOKS
AVAILABLE FROM PAN MACMILLAN

1-4050-6719-5	Reclaiming Desire	Dr Andrew Goldstein and Dr Marianne Branden	£12.99
1-4050-7759-x	Perfectly Normal	Dr Sandra Pertot	£10.99
1-4050-6726-8	Lasting Love	Gay Hendricks and Kathlyn Hendricks	£8.99
1-4050-6723-3	Everything You Need to Know About The Menopause	Ellen Phillips	£14.99
1-4050-7758-1	Healing Without Freud or Prozac	Dr David Servan–Schreiber	£7.99
1-4050-3340-1	When Your Body Gets the Blues	Marie-Annette Brown & Jo Robinson	£10.99

All Pan Macmillan titles can be ordered from our website, *www.panmacmillan.com*, or from your local bookshop and are also available by post from:

Bookpost, PO Box 29, Douglas, Isle of Man IM99 1BQ

Tel: 01624 677237; fax: 01624 670923; e-mail: *bookshop@enterprise.net*; or visit: *www.bookpost.co.uk*. Credit cards accepted. Free postage and packing in the United Kingdom

Prices shown above were correct at time of going to press.

Pan Macmillan reserve the right to show new retail prices on covers which may differ from those previously advertised in the text or elsewhere.

For information about buying *Rodale* titles in **Australia**, contact Pan Macmillan Australia. Tel: 1300 135 113; fax: 1300 135 103; e-mail: *customer.service@macmillan.com.au*; or visit: *www.panmacmillan.com.au*

For information about buying *Rodale* titles in **New Zealand**, contact Macmillan Publishers New Zealand Limited. Tel: (09) 414 0356; fax: (09) 414 0352; e-mail: *lyn@macmillan.co.nz*; or visit: *www.macmillan.co.nz*

For information about buying *Rodale* titles in **South Africa**, contact Pan Macmillan South Africa. Tel: (011) 325 5220; fax: (011) 325 5225; e-mail: *marketing@panmacmillan.co.za*

RODALE

MACMILLAN

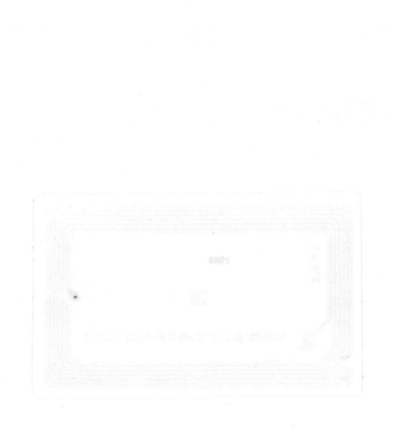

'There is a great deal of hard information for childless women – particularly those who can be helped by the new reproductive technologies – but there is very little understanding of the emotional difficulties of those who are childless, particularly in the long-term.

I hope this book will reach at least the family and friends of childless women – men included – because they often need an education in sympathy. In fact, I think all women would take something from it; it makes you ask what being a woman means.'

HILARY MANTEL, bestselling author

'The authors deal with all the issues one by one with admirable clarity and beguiling good sense. Their research is impeccable, and the authenticity of the personal stories painfully accurate. In the end, however, their mission is to help women realise that not having children can be every bit as positive as having a brood of six, and that childlessness need not mean a life without children. I was always aware that I was in the hands of two intelligent and thoughtful women who wanted to pool their own pain – and recovery from pain – for the benefit of women like me.'

DILLIE KEANE, writer, and co-founder of *Fascinating Aïda*

Even now, many women find it very difficult to discuss their childlessness with family and friends. This book offers support, shared experience and practical strategies to all those for whom childlessness is not a positive choice but a circumstance they have to learn to live with.

The authors have interviewed a large number of women for this book; their personal stories reflect the myriad reasons why women do not have children. Anyone who is learning to live with the fact that she may/will never have a child, or that having had one child she will never have another, will welcome this sensitive, practical and non-judgmental look at a profoundly complicated and personal issue.

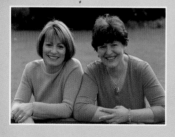

Rachel Black, left, runs her own market research consultancy, and Louise Scull, right, was, until recently, a banker. Both are childless.

MACMILLAN

RODALE

www.panmacmillan.com
£12.99

www.rodale.co.uk
Cover photograph: Corbis
Cover design: D. R. Ink

www.beyondchildlessness.com

ISBN 1-4050-7761-1

9 781405 077613